cooking your way to gorgeous

Skin-Friendly Superfoods, Age-Reversing Recipes, and Fabulous Homemade Facials

SCOTT-VINCENT BORBA

celebrity esthetician | nutraceutical expert

Health Communications, Inc.
Deerfield Beach, Florida

www.hcibooks.com

The information contained in this publication is not intended to replace the services of a physician, nor does it constitute a doctor-patient relationship. All content in this publication is provided for informational purposes, and readers should consult their own physicians concerning any recommendations. You should not use the information in this publication for diagnosing or treating a medical or health condition. If you have or suspect you have an urgent medical problem, promptly contact your professional healthcare provider. Any application of the suggestions in this publication is at the reader's discretion. All information is for educational purposes only and is not intended as medical advice, diagnosis, or prescription. When trying facials, to avoid any potential allergic reactions any time you make a facial mask, test it on the inside of your wrist first, before the mask touches your face. Most supermarkets label items with possible allergen-containing ingredients; however, there is always a risk of contamination. There is also a possibility that manufacturers of said commercial foods could change the formulation at any time, without notice. Readers concerned with food allergies need to be aware of this risk.

Neither Scott-Vincent Borba* nor Ali Morra-Pearlman assume any liability for adverse reactions to food consumed, or items one may come in contact with while trying recipes, hair treatments, and facials outlined in this book. Although most products used in hair treatments and facials are derived from natural products (fruits, vegetables, and so forth), every skin type is unique in its response to various vitamins and minerals, and the combinations thereof.

**Library of Congress Cataloging-in-Publication Data
is available through the Library of Congress.**

©2013 Scott-Vincent Borba

ISBN-13: 978-0-7573-1718-7
ISBN-10: 0-7573-1718-9

HCI, its logos, and its marks are trademarks of Health Communications, Inc.

Publisher: Health Communications, Inc.
      3201 S.W. 15th Street
      Deerfield Beach, FL 33442-8190

Cover photo of Scott-Vincent Borba by Kelsey Edwards Studios
Cover design by Larissa Hise Henoch
Interior design and formatting by Lawna Patterson Oldfield

This book is in loving memory of my beloved father and best friend Anthony R. Borba Sr., and my unstoppable beautiful mother Evelyn Ann Borba. I hope all that I do makes you proud and can be used as an example of how well you raised my siblings and me.

Without the support of my two incredible, stunning sisters, Stacy Ann Broderick and Sandra Ann Telfer, I wouldn't be able to create with courage! There have been many conversations in which you have told me to keep my blinders on and not worry about all the noise.

Thank you to my charitable partners, Covenant House and The Pancreatic Cancer Action Network for allowing me to herald your work and help try to advance your mission.

Without my faith in God, Jesus, and the Virgin Mother, I would be nothing. I'm humbled that I have the opportunity every day to work at the things that I love, which fuels my passion for helping others. I am grateful for the strength that the Holy Spirit provides me to keep pushing forward to seek my dreams. If my work were to make it to television, I could tell the world that my prayers had been heard. Why? Because I want to showcase that you can be God loving and a good example of hard work and still achieve huge success in an honest way.

This first ever inside-out beauty cookbook was inspired by my desire to change my own aesthetics in an innovative and fun way. I want to help answer your need for connecting with food as natural medicine to address skin, health, and beauty challenges. Please allow me to challenge you today to take ownership of your personal health and cook your way to a more gorgeous you from the inside out!

Besos,
Scott-Vincent Borba

Contents

Acknowledgments

Kelsey Edwards Studios for happening into my life! We met by forces of kismet and you will always be a part of my family. Thank you for shooting this cover and photographing many of my major events, modeling jobs, agency headshots, and important projects. You believed in me since I set foot in Los Angeles, and friends like you are hard to come by, indeed.

Frank Weinman, a terrific book agent who supported my creative ideas and never tried to change who I am.

Allison Janse for being the best publishing partner I could ever ask for. Thank you for not stifling my wacky innovations and for pushing me to be even more creative. You are patient and refreshing, and I'm blessed to be working with you on these last two projects and many more to come.

Eric J. Allen, a close friend (and willing guinea pig) who was there with me to test all my beauty concoctions, recipes, and products. Having one of the top celebrity makeup artists and my closest confidant by my side since we both started out in the industry has been a lifesaver. Thank you for all you have done, all the years of listening, and never once telling me that I couldn't accomplish my goals.

My writer Ali Morra-Pearlman who breathed life into my ideas with her wonderful way of language and originality. A great partner for the world's first ever beauty cookbook! What a fun and challenging adventure we went on with this project. You are extremely talented, and I'm proud to call you my great friend and colleague.

Valerie Castro for your exceptional eye and constant cheerleading! You picked me up many a day when I needed the support to push forward. You are a special person and a wonderful source of guidance.

Friends and supporters like Nancy O'Dell, Angela Basset, Selena Gomez, Stacy Keebler, CS Lee, and Jennifer Love Hewitt (among many others). You trust in my expertise and I can't thank you enough for showcasing my philosophy of inside-out beauty as realistically as humanly possible—on your skin!

Mi otra familia. I love our virtual chats and seeing your faces and friendly messages daily. You are my tabula rasa, and without you I wouldn't be inspired to keep innovating products. I constantly have you in the back of my mind when I create or push myself to achieve a higher goal. I always ask, *can I honor you with this effort and make you proud?* You are my engine and my magic and I appreciate you tremendously. *Nos vemos en el cyberspace! Besos.*

Introduction: Eat Your Way to Gorgeous Skin

All of us are looking to spend less but still get high-level results with our beauty routines. The good news is that including foods in your diet that support healthy skin is easier and more cost effective than any other skin-care method. Feeding your skin from the inside out with skin-friendly foods and whipping up skin-saving beauty treatments with things you have in your pantry are what I call being *skin savvy*. What many people don't know is that your kitchen pantry holds many secret ingredients with multiple uses that will give you skin-revitalizing results. I will show you how to use many of them, such as olive oil, baking soda, honey, canned beans, avocados, vanilla extract, sea salt, oatmeal, and fiber powder, and I will also introduce you to many new powerful ingredient favorites.

If you choose to live life productively and to the max, if you are open to lifestyle improvement, achieving better skin quickly, a slimmer silhouette, and a pared-down medicine cabinet, plus fewer trips to the cosmetics counter, this book is for you. Enjoy it over the course of many months, or years, and I guarantee you'll see and feel a significant difference. *Cooking Your Way to Gorgeous* teaches you how to combine the power of ingestible nutrients and topical ingredients to visibly change the appearance of your skin.

You will read a lot about "hero" ingredients in this book. When discussing gorgeous skin, the term pops up frequently. A hero is any nutrient or food, or combination thereof, that boosts health, wellness, and beauty. Hero ingredients and recipes offer you A+ benefits, above and beyond the rest. You'll notice that we have labeled quite a few recipes in this book as "hero recipes"—these are my all-time favorites and most efficacious. In the

1

chapters that follow, I will explain what these hero foods can do for your skin and offer you a wealth of simple, delicious recipes you can make with them.

But for now, here is your jump-start cheat sheet: The most important hero foods to eat, in my opinion, are:

1) berries, camu camu, and pomegranates (antioxidants)
2) seeds, nuts, and sprouts (protein and vitamin E)
3) fish (omega-3 fatty acids)
4) greens, the darker the better (vitamin A)
5) whole grains (antioxidants)

These hero foods work for every body part and physical channel to provide internal and external beauty. In this book, I encourage you to not only cook with hero items to *feed your skin,* but to use them in facial recipes and concoctions to *apply to* your *skin.*

Focusing on beauty as a whole, this book will help you leverage your everyday eating habits to become the most beautiful person you can be inside and out. You can get a skin-care guru, health and beauty coach, and a personal chef without the $2,000 per hour price tag. I'm all about the pep talk and helping YOU reach your goals. If you like chocolate, you will get it. Craving nachos? I have a recipe that's good for your skin and cheesy delicious. Are you a hearty-soup fan or a burger connoisseur? In this book you will find simple, fresh recipes that can actually aid you in your quest for clearer skin. If you like your mac and cheese and cake, too, you will have them—with a high performance twist that's beneficial to your skin and beauty. Even your cocktails get a Borba health boost, as was written about in the *New York Times.* I want you to use all the information I have researched, reviewed, and refined over the years so you don't have to reinvent the way you cook. I want you to look and feel your best without having to sacrifice what you love to eat. Eating the foods you love in the *right way* will reveal your healthiest skin. When you look great you feel great, your inner light shines through, your beauty beams across the room, and that shining inner beauty conquers all.

If you are serious about improving the health and appearance of your skin, this cooking beauty book is for you. In these user-friendly recipes, the key ingredients can also be used to create homemade facials or cosmetic tricks while you prepare the meal, or during the few minutes you sneak for yourself in your own home spa.

Each ingredient can yield multiple uses for total body benefit. For example, due to their high vitamin C content, red and green hot chile peppers and bell peppers can power your skin to glow. Making a great chicken sauté with these ingredients, plus grapeseed oil for the pan, will give you multiple health and beauty benefits in one fell swoop, *deliciously*. But did you also know that when you apply hot chile peppers on your skin it helps with circulation, which is great for dimply skin on the legs, tummy, and body? A quick, targeted body serum would be to muddle (mash/mix together) the chile pepper or a chile paste along with the grapeseed oil and rub it vigorously on the skin before a hot shower. Wash it off when you feel the tingle.

If you have a lot on your plate, and you don't have the time or focus to radically change the way you cook, eat, and care for your skin (who does?) but you are open to improvement—this book gives you an easy route to beautiful skin. It's the insider's scoop on how to achieve results *without* completely overhauling your eating habits or lifestyle—and it's immensely helpful and fun, too. You will find time-saving tips, tricks, fun facts, home-spa treatments, and problem-solving food ingredients that are essential for increased energy and improved health—and will help the body and complexion at any age.

For example, do you ever find that when bedtime rolls around that you and your loved one retire at the same time, but, by the time you've just gotten into your beauty routine, your partner's already done and fast asleep in bed? You dab on cream for that dry patch, and astringent for that breakout, a dab of moisturizer A for the forehead, a slathering of moisturizer B for the neck . . . pimple cream on the left, vitamin E on the scar, a pat-pat under the jowls for tightening (doesn't work), serum on the nose, cream under the eyes, Vaseline on your lips, skin brightening cream on your cheeks . . . too much time spent catering to bathroom-business minutia is eating up your free time! This is precious time you could be reading, relaxing in front of the TV, or, *ahem*, enjoying your partner. Wouldn't it be fabulous if you could pare down your beauty rituals and synthesize your facial products and procedures? If you had better skin overall, you could. And you will, if you can tweak the way you eat.

As you begin your journey, the biggest thing to know is that even if you start to revert to your old habits—unhealthy eating can be a vicious cycle—you can quickly make up for lost time and get back on track, so don't give up! Simply by being mindful, you can control and nurture your beauty. You will learn how to experiment with items you already have at home to make your own regimen, meal, or skin-care items on the cheap. For example, if you use topical anti-aging serums or even basic moisturizers, why wouldn't you use the same *active ingredients* internally? This book will give you the tools to creatively synergize both the topical and internal systems to work together. For example, if you get great results from a skin-care product that contains vitamin C, I will show you how to get optimal results by making recipes that contain vitamin C. If you're using an ingredient in a topical skin-care product, try to eat foods that contain the same ingredients.

What you do and don't have in your cabinets, pantry, and refrigerator will help keep your skin looking its best. With over 125 healthy recipes, quick and easy facials, hair-care treatments, and pantry-stocking tips, curbing the frenzied cycle of unhealthy eating and recapturing your beauty power will be an eye opener, a game changer, and won't dent your dollars. Many of us suffer from acne scarring, premature gray hair, smoker's face, unwanted facial hair, dark under-eye circles . . . but let's face it, that's just the tip of the iceberg. Dry sensitive skin, enlarged pores, bacne, wrinkles, weight challenges . . . whatever your challenge, *Cooking Your Way to Gorgeous* will help keep skin looking flawlessly translucent and radiant. I want you to feel enthralled, to walk away looking and feeling gorgeous—and empowered inside and out. You should feel inspired by your own health and life!

—Scott-Vincent Borba

Take It from the Top

Chapter 1

Your hair is the frame of your face. Hair makes a statement that dictates a lot about your personality, too. When it looks great you feel confident and beautiful. When it looks dry, frizzy, or oily, you pull it back in a ponytail or smother it under a hat. Good news: It's very easy to enhance and improve your hair's beautiful luster and shine and fall in love with it all over again. Square one: Make sure that you are drinking at least eight 8-ounce glasses of water daily. Not only will your skin repair and recharge, but your entire body will thank you, including your hair. If you find the taste of water to be boring—and lots of people do—squeeze in some lemon juice, use the flavored water brand of your choice, or turn your water into a pitcher of cold, easy-to-gulp green tea. Green tea may influence the serum levels of certain hormones that are linked to at least one form of hair loss common in women and men.

To have radiant, healthy, and glowing skin and full, shiny hair, it's important to understand that skin and hair share the same nutritional requirements. In other words, if your body is healthy and nourished, your hair will shine and your skin will glow, too.

Since many of us can't afford frequent salon visits or high-end designer shampoos, I will give you some recipes for homemade hair treatments.

TIP: Give your skin an antioxidant boost by treating yourself to a green tea Popsicle. Brew a quart of green tea. Once it has cooled, add in ¼ cup Truvia Baking Blend, and stir until dissolved. Transfer to Popsicle molds and freeze.

And speaking of shampoos, when you read the labels, try to avoid products with fillers such as mineral oil and petrolatum. These products clog hair follicles, inhibiting hair growth. They also sit on top of the hair blocking needed moisture from entering the hair shaft. You want products that give moisture and contain protein to keep the hair strong.

More important, to keep your hair its healthiest you need to know how to boost its nutrients *internally* to nourish hair inside out. Try to eat foods with iron, B vitamins, and antioxidants—the nutrients that are essential for hair growth and repair—as well as biotin, which makes the body produce extra keratin. Keratin is the protein that forms the chemical base for hair and nails. The human body is not capable of producing its own antioxidants; therefore, we must incorporate antioxidants into our diet and onto our hair and skin. This chapter will give you the best heroes for hair with the highest food nutrients that help provide inside-out benefits. You will also get tips that can help get you started on reclaiming your confident glow. Review the recipes, see what their benefits are, and make a hair-care treatment using some of those ingredients. Cooking for beauty benefits from the inside out is the modern approach to beauty and a central benefit of *Cooking Your Way to Gorgeous*. In this chapter and throughout the book you will find that many recipes incorporate fruits and vegetables, the most excellent source of natural antioxidants available to us, and that many of these recipes contain ingredients that are bursting with benefits for beauty as a whole.

Supplementing a few key ingredients into your snacking habits and meals will help your hair shine and flow no matter its style, length, cut, or color. These active ingredients are essential for hair gloss, growth, and strength. I want you to celebrate and embrace your 'do, down to its last little quirk!

My goal for you is that by the time you reach the end of this chapter, you have a new source for recipes and hair-health information. If you try a handful of these recipes and at-home spa treatments you will surely start to notice improvements in your hair and scalp, among other total body benefits. Bookmark, dog-ear, highlight, circle, or snapshot the ones that work best for you and pass them on.

TOP 5
Hero Foods for
Hair and Scalp Health

Eggs—a rich source of biotin, key for hair strength and growth.

Salmon—a biotin-rich protein source.

Walnuts—a good source of biotin, also contain omega-3s, which support scalp health and give hair a healthy, shiny appearance.

Spinach—this green contains vitamins A and C, which help your body produce sebum, a natural scalp oil that moisturizes hair and combats dryness.

Gelatin (or pectin, if you are vegan)—a fabulous ingredient for shine and moisture lock.

GRILLED SALMON with GINGER GLAZE

Makes 4 Servings

A hhh, the benefits of salmon. I think if I were stuck on a desert island with only a few foods to sustain me, salmon would be one I would choose for the long haul. The high protein content in salmon helps with hair health. The omega-3s found in salmon lock moisture into skin cells, encouraging the production of strong collagen and elastin fibers, which contribute to more youthful looking skin. Omega-3s have also been known to alleviate skin blemishes while providing nourishment to hair follicles, helping hair grow healthy and preventing hair loss. A rich supply of proteins is also important for hair growth.

Ingredients:

4 (8-ounce) fresh salmon fillets
   —superb protein!

Salt, to taste

⅓ cup cold water

¼ cup seasoned rice vinegar

2 tablespoons brown sugar

1 tablespoon hot chile paste
   —can help with weight loss

1 tablespoon finely grated fresh ginger

4 cloves garlic, minced

1 teaspoon soy sauce—iodine source

¼ cup chopped fresh basil

Preparation:

1 Preheat the grill on medium heat and lightly oil the grate with cooking spray.

2 Season the salmon fillets with salt.

3 Combine the water, rice vinegar, brown sugar, chile paste, ginger, garlic, and soy sauce in a small saucepan over medium heat. Bring the mixture to a boil, reduce the heat to medium, and simmer until barely thickened, about 2 minutes.

4 Place the salmon on the preheated grill; cook for 6 to 8 minutes per side, or until the fish flakes easily with a fork.

5 Sprinkle the basil on top of the salmon; top with the ginger glaze.

WILD-CAUGHT ALASKAN SALMON
with TOMATO SALSA

<u>Makes 2 Servings</u>

Like many of us these days, I am leaning more toward the consumption of organic foods in my home, and in my cleaning products, too. (I've been trying to "go green" for years.) This awareness incorporates yet another arena of thinking when it comes to fish—wild-caught or farm-raised? Most of the salmon consumed nowadays is farm-raised. I will leave it to you to make your own informed decisions about what is right for your needs and budget, but for this recipe I encourage you to go for the slightly more expensive wild-caught Alaskan salmon so you can maximize its health benefits. Food is like medicine, so you want to always be putting good food in to avoid the medicine later! Fresh wild Alaskan salmon is an extremely powerful anti-aging food.

Ingredients: Salmon

1½ pounds salmon filet cut into 4 pieces, skin and bones removed
1 tablespoon lemon juice
Salt and pepper, to taste

Salsa

1 large ripe tomato, seeds and excess pulp removed, diced small
3 tablespoons finely minced onion
3 medium cloves garlic, pressed
1 to 2 tablespoons jalapeño pepper—antioxidants; vitamins A and C
1 tablespoon minced fresh ginger
1 tablespoon coarsely chopped pumpkin seeds—superfood
¼ cup chopped fresh cilantro
2 tablespoons lemon juice
1 tablespoon extra-virgin olive oil
Salt and pepper, to taste

Preparation: Salmon

1 To quick-broil: preheat the broiler on high and place a cast-iron skillet under the heat for about 10 minutes to get it very hot. The pan should be 5 to 7 inches from the heat source.

2 Rub the salmon with the lemon juice and a little salt and pepper.

3 Using an oven mitt, pull the skillet away from the heat and place the salmon in it skin-side down. Return the skillet to the broiler. The salmon will cook rapidly on both sides so it will be done quickly, in about 7 minutes, depending on its thickness (figure 10 minutes for every inch of thickness). Salmon is best when it's still pink inside and will flake easily when it's cooked.

Salsa

Combine all the salsa ingredients and mix well with a large spoon. Top the salsa over the salmon and enjoy.

Why Salmon Is So Good

One 4-ounce portion of salmon contains at least 2 grams of omega-3 fats—more than the average U.S. adult gets over the course of several days. Omega-3s also help lubricate the intestinal walls, allowing toxins in your body to be absorbed by the oils. Salmon contains small bioactive protein peptides that may provide special support for joint cartilage, insulin effectiveness, and control of inflammation in the digestive tract.

TIP: You can use an omega-3 fish oil capsule right now. Take one capsule and pierce it with a needle. Squeeze out the gel and use it around the eye area and on the face as a concentrated omega-3 serum.

KOREAN OMELET

Makes 2 Servings

Kye-ran-mari *in Korean translates as* kye-ran, *meaning "egg" and* mari *meaning "rolled." And since I'm all about extrapolating beauty tips and interesting information from all over the world, I recommend this rolled egg dish. This unique alternative to everyday scrambled eggs or cheese omelets offers the benefits of copper from sesame, iodine from nori (a sea vegetable or "seaweed"), and of course protein from the eggs. This is one of my favorite omelets.*

Ingredients:

4 eggs—keratin source

3 tablespoons water

1 tablespoon soy sauce

1 tablespoon sesame seeds
  —copper and manganese source

½ tablespoon peanut oil

½ sheet nori, julienned—nori, known
  as "the reservoir of vitamins," contains
  12 different vitamins and as much
  protein as soybeans

Preparation:

1 Beat the eggs together with all the ingredients, except for the peanut oil and nori.

2 Heat the peanut oil in a large skillet on medium.

3 Cook the egg mixture on one side like an omelet, until almost done; the inside should still be a bit runny.

4 Sprinkle the nori along one side. Roll up like a jellyroll and cut in half to serve.

 Limp Hair Treatment

Try this while you're cooking or when you have some me-time before your shower: Whip up 3 to 4 egg whites in a blender until foamy. Place them on your scalp for 30 minutes only. Rinse and style for a great root lift for limp hair.

 TIP: Seafood and seaweed are rich natural sources of iodine, which prevents hair from drying out.

MAPLE SCRAMBLED EGGS
and TURKEY BACON

Makes 2 Servings

If you, like me, enjoy the flavors of sweet and savory in the same dish, then you will enjoy this all-American breakfast packed with energy. Maple syrup is highly moisturizing for hair, and eggs are excellent sources of hair-growth-boosting biotin.

Ingredients:

2 slices turkey bacon—lower in fat than regular bacon

2 whole eggs—protein

4 egg whites—protein with less cholesterol

2 teaspoons warm maple syrup—antioxidant source

Preparation:

1 Coat a small skillet with canola oil spray and preheat over medium heat. Add the turkey bacon to the skillet and cook until crispy, about 1 minute per side.

2 Transfer the bacon to a paper towel–covered plate (to absorb grease), and return the skillet to the burner.

3 In a small bowl, whip together the whole egg and egg whites. Add the eggs to the skillet and scramble. Cook for about two minutes, then crumble the bacon and add it to the eggs; continue to scramble the eggs until cooked through.

4 Transfer the eggs to a plate and drizzle the maple syrup on top.

 Maple Syrup Hair Treatment for Dry Hair

You will need 5 tablespoons of pure maple syrup and 1 tablespoon of honey. Heat the ingredients in the microwave for about 15 seconds. Place an old towel over your shoulders. Remove the syrup/honey mix from microwave, wait until it cools, and then apply it to dry hair, focusing on the ends, and comb through it with a wide-toothed comb to spread it evenly. Cover your head with a shower cap. Let the treatment sit for 20 minutes. Rinse it off in the shower and shampoo as normal.

2-MINUTE EGG SOUFFLÉ

Makes 1 Serving

*T*his basic dish could look like it was served up from your quaint corner bistro, but in fact it's the microwaving process that makes the eggs rise and look prize-worthy. Eggs and egg whites are excellent sources of protein, and they promote healthy hair and nails because of their high sulfur content and wide array of vitamins and minerals. Many people find their hair growing faster after adding eggs to their diet. Salsa contains nothing but good-for-you ingredients and, therefore, is a terrific condiment that's got some bulk to it, maximum taste, and minimal calories.

Ingredients:

1 egg

2 egg whites

1 tablespoon medium-hot salsa, brand of your choice or homemade
—a calorie watcher's best friend

2 shakes Tabasco sauce—capsaicin, a natural metabolism booster

Preparation:

1 Spray a small microwave-safe bowl with canola oil spray. Crack the egg and egg whites into the bowl and whip together with a fork. (Hang on tight, the bowl edges might be slippery from the cooking spray.)

2 Add 1 heaping tablespoon of salsa and a squirt of hot sauce to the egg mix, if desired. Mix well. Microwave for 2 minutes, or until the egg is just cooked through.

TIP: Do a fresh test on your eggs before you cook with them. Gently drop an egg in water. If it sinks, it's fresh—perfect for soufflés and poaching. If it stays submerged with its wide end up, it's older but good for most uses. If it floats, throw it away.

 Olive Oil Hair Mask for Scalp Hydration

Blend 4 tablespoons olive oil and 2 whole eggs together thoroughly. Apply mixture to the scalp and massage in evenly. Cover hair with a plastic shower cap or plastic wrap. Let set for 10 minutes and wash hair as usual.

RUSSIAN EGG and MUSHROOM SALAD

Makes 2 to 3 Servings

*T*his recipe does not require eggs from Russia (although wouldn't it be kind of neat if it did?). Russian egg refers to a style of egg preparation. In this case, it is hard-boiled with specific ingredients that are akin to the deviled- or picnic-egg category.

Ingredients:

5 tablespoons canola oil

1 pound mushrooms, roughly chopped—potassium source; very low cal

½ medium yellow onion, roughly chopped

⅓ cup finely chopped fresh dill—contains essential oils

4 hard-boiled eggs, roughly chopped

¾ cup mayonnaise

2 tablespoons Dijon mustard

1 or 2 tablespoons fresh lemon juice—vitamin C

Kosher salt, to taste

Freshly ground black pepper, to taste

4 slices whole wheat bread

Preparation:

1 Heat 3 tablespoons of the oil in a 10- or 12-inch skillet over medium-high heat, and add the mushrooms. Cook, stirring often, until lightly browned, 14 to 16 minutes. Transfer to a large bowl, and set aside. Wipe out the skillet.

2 Heat the remaining oil in the skillet over medium-high heat, and add the onion. Cook, stirring often, until the onions begin to soften; then reduce the heat to low and continue to cook until lightly caramelized, 10 to 15 minutes. Transfer to the bowl with the mushrooms. Add the dill and eggs, and stir to mix.

3 In a small bowl, whisk together the mayonnaise, mustard, and lemon juice. Add a couple of spoonfuls to the mushroom mixture, and toss until evenly combined. Taste, and add more dressing as needed.

4 Season to taste with salt, pepper, and lemon juice.

5 Serve on lightly toasted wheat bread.

HIJIKI RICE SALAD

Makes 6 to 8 Servings

*T*his is one of my favorite appetizers when I go out for Japanese food. I had to frequent the same restaurant for almost two years before the chef would share his recipe with me! Like nori, hijiki is a type of sea vegetable. When hijiki is reconstituted it looks like black noodles. It's a traditional Japanese food that's been a part of their balanced diet for centuries, probably because it's low in calories and fat and contains fiber, iron, and a good balance of calcium and magnesium. You can even sprinkle it dry into salads to add a dash of salty flavor and a dose of calcium. The Japanese believe that eating hijiki will yield thick lustrous hair, and they should know—arigato!

Ingredients:

½ ounce dried hijiki seaweed (about ½ cup)

1¼ cups water

⅓ teaspoon iodized salt

½ cup uncooked long grain brown rice—fiber source; easily digestible
   if you are gluten intolerant; economical; good shelf life

1 tablespoon sesame seeds

2 scallions, finely chopped

¾ cup snow peas, cut into thin strips—natural fat burner; excellent
   source of vitamins A and C

1 small carrot, grated

½ teaspoon grated fresh ginger

1 ounce brown rice vinegar—contains 20 amino acids

½ teaspoon honey (or use vegan sugar or honey substitute)

1 tablespoon olive oil

Freshly ground black pepper, optional

Preparation:

1 Soak hijiki in cool water for 1 hour, then drain. Notice how it doubles
   in size and weight.

2 Bring the water and salt to a boil in a medium saucepan; add the rice.
   Turn the heat down to low and cover, simmering the rice for about
   20 minutes.

3 While the rice simmers, cook the hijiki: In a saucepan, cover it generously with water. Simmer it over medium-low heat for about 15 minutes, or until hijiki is tender. Strain and rinse under cold water.

4 Toast the sesame seeds in a small, dry skillet over medium heat, shaking the pan occasionally, until the seeds brown lightly. Move the seeds to a plate to cool.

5 Mix the scallions, snow peas, and carrots in a large bowl.

6 Combine the ginger, vinegar, honey, and oil in a small bowl, whisking to mix into a vinaigrette.

7 Add the warm cooked rice to the vegetables. Add the cool hijiki and the vinaigrette. Toss well; add the sesame seeds and pepper, if using. Toss again.

8 Serve the salad warm, or chill it for 1 hour first. It will keep in the fridge, covered, for up to 3 days.

OYSTERS BORBA

*S*lurp to beauty with this option for the oyster curious! Buy oysters fresh from your local fish market. Oysters contain two amino acids that are said to raise levels of the sex hormones testosterone and estrogen. Low fat, zinc-loaded for hair health, and functional! Dig in.

Ingredients:

2 tablespoons olive oil

2 tablespoons all-purpose flour

¼ cup water

2 cups wilted and chopped spinach—phytonutrients

½ cup chopped fresh basil

3 cloves garlic, minced—intense heart helper

Juice and zest of 1 large lemon

½ teaspoon hot sauce

1 pinch kosher salt

Ground black pepper, to taste

24 large fresh oysters, with juice, tightly closed in shell

2 tablespoons grated Parmesan cheese

Preparation:

1 In a small skillet, heat the oil over medium heat. Add the flour and cook 3 to 4 minutes, stirring continuously until a thick, smooth paste forms. Remove from the heat and add the water, spinach, basil, garlic, lemon juice and zest, and hot sauce. Whisk quickly until a thick sauce forms. Season with salt and pepper to taste.

2 Preheat the oven to 400°F. Shuck the oysters, reserving the shells. Put one oyster per shell in the deepest reserved half-shells. Top with a spoonful of the spinach mixture and sprinkle with the Parmesan.

3 Place the half-shells on a baking sheet covered with aluminum foil and carefully place in the oven. Bake for 8 to 10 minutes, until the oysters are cooked inside, the filling begins to brown, and the oysters are no longer translucent but still tender. Serve immediately.

ISRAELI COUSCOUS SALAD
with PAPRIKA

*Y*ou don't have to travel far to get a taste of the Old World with this simple side dish. Couscous [koos-koos] is light and tasty, a good-for-you grain pasta with lots of fiber and selenium, too.

Ingredients: Dressing

⅓ cup extra-virgin olive oil

2 tablespoons white balsamic vinegar

2 teaspoons paprika—contains vitamin C and capsaicin, a powerful anti-inflammatory for skin and body

1 teaspoon kosher salt

½ teaspoon freshly ground black pepper

Couscous

1 tablespoon extra-virgin olive oil

8 ounces Israeli couscous

½ teaspoon kosher salt

2 cups coarsely chopped, packed baby spinach leaves—higher in nutrient content than virtually any other food

12 ounces (about 2 cups) grape or cherry tomatoes—low-cal superfruits

4 ounces (about 1 cup) feta cheese, coarsely crumbled or chopped into ½-inch pieces

1 cup coarsely chopped, jarred red bell peppers, drained

½ cup chopped, fresh, flat-leaf parsley—vitamin K helps diminish bruises, scratches, and stretch marks

⅓ cup slivered almonds, toasted—protein

¼ cup chopped fresh mint

Kosher salt and freshly ground black pepper, to taste

Preparation: Dressing

Whisk the oil, vinegar, paprika, salt, and pepper in a small bowl until smooth.

Preparation: Couscous

1 Heat the oil over medium-high heat in a large saucepan. Cook the couscous in the oil, stirring frequently, until golden, 4 to 5 minutes. Add 2 cups of water and the salt and bring to a boil. Reduce the heat to medium-low. Cover and simmer until the couscous is just tender and the liquid is absorbed, 9 to 10 minutes. Set aside to cool slightly.

2 Mix together the spinach, tomatoes, cheese, peppers, parsley, almonds, and mint in a large bowl. Add the couscous and the dressing. Toss until all the ingredients are coated. Salt and pepper, to taste. Transfer to a large serving bowl and serve.

TIP: If you like the look of a suntan but have sworn off those damaging rays, you can mix iodine with your moisturizer to increase skin color and glow. If you opt for a shimmery moisturizer, you're ready for a night on the town.

WARM ORZO PASTA SALAD

*O*rzo is a small pasta that resembles grains of rice. Orzo dishes can be quite dense, as the pasta will compact into a solid mass when cooked. Orzo is a low-fat food high in iron and fiber. This recipe also calls for a generous helping of spinach, which is a powerhouse of nutrients. Among vegetables, spinach contains the most protein! And cooking it releases beta-carotene and lutein, which your scalp and hair need for health, glow, and strength.

Ingredients:

6 ounces orzo (about 1 cup)

⅓ cup chopped onion

1 clove garlic, minced

2 tablespoons olive oil

7 cups baby spinach (about 6 ounces)

⅓ cup chopped black olives—helps smooth skin

½ teaspoon salt

¼ teaspoon black pepper

1½ cups halved grape tomatoes

2 teaspoons lemon juice

¼ cup soft goat (chèvre) cheese—calcium

Preparation:

1 Boil the orzo according to package directions. Drain and set aside.

2 Sauté the onion and garlic in oil in a skillet over medium-low heat until softened. Add the spinach and olives and turn the spinach with tongs until just wilted, about 1 minute. Add the salt and pepper.

3 Add the orzo to the spinach mixture along with the tomatoes and lemon juice. Toss and season to taste with salt and pepper. Serve with small dollops of goat cheese on top.

POMEGRANATE BERRY JELL-O

Makes One 12-Cup Mold

*H*ello, Jell-O! Where have you been? Getting a dose of gelatin in your diet is great for increasing the shine in your hair. In addition to a host of benefits, gelatin is known to keep hair healthy and to help hair grow stronger, faster, and longer. Using gelatin as a major dietary protein is an easy way to restrict the amino acids that are associated with many of the problems of aging, too. The high amounts of protein in Jell-O are what work the wonders. Your hair will start to look glossier and healthier within weeks of eating gelatin on a regular basis. It's a great dessert that's virtually fat free. If you don't feel like making this delicious recipe every time your hair needs a boost, you have my blessing to buy Jell-O straight off the shelf, or simply try the Gelatin/Pectin Hair Mask instead.

Ingredients:

4 envelopes unflavored gelatin powder or pectin—my preference
   —right next to gelatin in the Jell-O aisle. (Pectin is made of plant
   solubles that mimic the consistency of gelatin.)
½ cup cold water
4 cups boiling pomegranate juice—antioxidant rich for heart health
3 cups ginger ale
2 cups mixed fresh blueberries and strawberries

Preparation:

1 In a bowl, sprinkle the gelatin evenly over the water and allow the gelatin to absorb the water for 2 minutes.

2 Add the boiling pomegranate juice to the gelatin mixture and stir until the gelatin is fully dissolved.

3 Stir in the ginger ale, transfer to a mold, and refrigerate until just thickened but not set. Be sure to be mindful of how much time the mold is chilling down—you don't want it to harden yet....

4 Fold the berries into the mold. Return to the refrigerator and let it set overnight.

Gelatin/Pectin Hair Mask

Mix together 1 tablespoon of unflavored gelatin, 1 cup of water, and 1 teaspoon of cider vinegar. Massage the gel-like mixture through shampooed hair and leave on for 5 minutes, then rinse. Great for fighting frizz.

PRO TIP

After applying hair masks or leave-in conditioners, wrap your hair with plastic wrap. It locks in moisture, helping to repair hair by smoothing hair cuticles. Try it!

How to Get Your Gelatin (and Collagen, Too)!

Gelatin is made up of collagen. That's right, collagen. It is derived from gelatin-rich bony and cartilaginous bits of animals. (Sorry, that's the reality.) Gelatin exists in the tough, gristly, bony cuts of meat like oxtails, lamb shanks, pork neck bones, and chicken wings, and also in skin. Long, slow, moist cooking turns these meat cuts silky and succulent, with incredible flavor. Even pork rinds are a terrific source of gelatin! You've heard of collagen cream, right? You may have even splurged on a jar of it, or been talked into buying it at the cosmetics counter, or convinced by your esthetician to try the "collagen facial." Well, the molecules in these creams are actually too big to penetrate the skin when applied topically. (Sorry, that's the reality, too.) On the other hand, taking collagen internally is immensely helpful.

APPLE PIE PITAS with WALNUTS

*A*n easy treat to assemble, no cooking required, and rich in vitamin E. *Walnuts provide heart-healthy monounsaturated fats and omega-3s, which help to keep your hair shiny and your scalp from drying to the point of flaking. Walnuts are a great "grab food" for a quick healthy snack. In this recipe, you also get the benefit of wheat germ, an excellent source of fiber. Wheat germ is near flavorless and makes for a wonderful healthy add-in to virtually any recipe. Wheat germ also adds an extra bit of crunch. You also get the benefit of flaxseed, also known as linseed, a reddish brown seed that's full of alpha-linoleic acid, a type of omega-3.*

Ingredients:

¼ cup cream cheese

2 teaspoons chopped walnuts,

1 teaspoon ground flaxseeds

2 tablespoons wheat germ

4 teaspoons chopped apple—leave skin on for added fiber

1 teaspoon cinnamon—antibacterial properties

3 teaspoons raisins or craisins

4 mini whole wheat pitas

Preparation:

Mix cream cheese, walnuts, flaxseed, wheat germ, apple, raisins or craisins, and cinnamon in a bowl. Stuff mixture inside pitas. Eat immediately.

Eat Your Wheat-ies!

The vitamins in wheat germ promote healthy hair growth and prevent split ends and other damage. Wheat germ is a powerful antioxidant full of high levels of vitamin E, which is an essential component in the growth of hair from the follicle. I love wheat germ sprinkled on ice cream—my friend's kids call them "crunchies"—because I know I am getting health benefits with my dessert. Wheat germ can also be used on top of a pizza, or in any pasta sauce without kids, or spouses, knowing.

ALMOND BUTTER and BANANA BLAST

*T*his is a quick-prep snack that's the perfect combination of protein, fat, and complex carbohydrates. The almond butter is high in nutritional value, loaded with protein and omega-3s that help sustain energy and concentration. The banana adds that touch of sweetness you crave and the potassium-rich density to make this a filling snack. You can also use almond butter and bananas as home-spa hair treatments—see recipes that follow.

Ingredients:

1 teaspoon salted almond butter

1 slice sprouted raisin bread, toasted—flourless

½ banana, sliced—potassium

Drizzle of honey

Sprinkle of cinnamon—skin-care benefits

½ teaspoon ground flaxseed

Preparation:

Spread the almond butter on the raisin bread. Top with the sliced bananas. Drizzle on the honey; sprinkle with cinnamon and the ground flaxseeds.

 Home-Spa Almond Butter Conditioning Hair Mask

After washing hair, slather it with almond butter and wait for at least 15 to 20 minutes before washing it off. The natural oils in almond butter will leave your hair soft and shiny.

 Home-Spa Banana Mask for Dry Hair

Combine 1 mashed banana, 1 egg, 3 tablespoons of honey, 3 tablespoons of milk, and 5 tablespoons of olive oil in a bowl. Using a wide-toothed comb, apply the mask to your hair from the roots to the ends. Let the mask soak in for about 15 to 30 minutes. If your hair is very damaged, leave the mask on longer. Rinse it out with cold water, then shampoo and condition as usual.

EASY GUACAMOLE

*O*ne *avocado contains about 29 grams of fat. This high-fat content can moisturize and nourish your hair, providing it with essential oils and moisturizers. Avocados are my favorite. I eat one whole avocado every day. You are doing great things for your hair and skin with every avo you eat. While very high in the right kind of dietary fat, they contain no cholesterol, have potassium and B vitamins, protein, and moisturizing properties that are great for hair health.*

Ingredients:

2 ripe avocados, peeled and pits removed—elixir of hair health
1 small onion, peeled and minced
1 clove garlic, peeled and minced—can help fight hair loss
1 small tomato, chopped
1½ tablespoons lime juice, or juice of 1 fresh lime—packed with vitamin C,
    important for immune system
Salt and pepper, to taste
Paprika to taste—antioxidant

Preparation:

Mash the avocado in a bowl, then stir in the remaining ingredients, except for the paprika. Sprinkle the paprika on top.

Serve cold with blue corn tortilla chips, or the chips of your preference.

 Avocado Hair Conditioner for All Hair Types

You'll need 1 avocado, 1 egg yolk, and 2 tablespoons of coconut milk. Cut the avocado in half, remove the skin and pit, and put the avocado in the blender. Using egg yolk only, add it to the blender with the coconut milk and blend until smooth. Wet hair and apply the mixture from the roots to the ends. Put a shower cap on over your hair to trap heat and to allow the conditioner to penetrate into your hair. Leave the conditioner on your hair for a minimum of 20 minutes or overnight. If you are short on time, apply blow-dryer heat to the shower cap. The longer you leave the conditioner on, the deeper its effects will be.

Avocado Hair Mask for Split Ends

An avocado mask can help moisturize and repair destroyed hair. Mix together 1 mashed avocado, ¼ cup of honey, and 1 can of coconut milk in a bowl. Put the mixture on *dry* hair, especially over split ends. Cover with a shower cap and blast the hair dryer over it for 5 minutes. Let the mask sit for an additional 30 minutes. Rinse well, but don't shampoo! This treatment will work toward giving you healthier hair overall.

 ### Mashed Avocado Treatment for Frizzy Hair

Mash half an avocado and massage it into clean, damp hair. Amp up the moisturizing by combining the avocado with 1 to 2 tablespoons of mayonnaise, which is a hydrating ingredient. Let it sit for 30 minutes before rinsing it out with shampoo.

 ### Turn Dull Hair to Dazzling

Mix together 2 tablespoons of extra-virgin olive, 1 ripe mashed avocado for added shine, and 1 tablespoon of mayonnaise. Spread through hair. Leave on for 10 minutes maximum. Rinse thoroughly. You can do this treatment up to once a week.

COCONUT RICE TO DIE FOR

Makes 4 Servings

A simple, secret family recipe that I want to share with you, this rice is rich and delicious, offering hair and scalp benefits from the coconut.

Ingredients:

2 cups rice

1½ cups light coconut milk

1 teaspoon grated fresh ginger—circulatory properties for scalp stimulation

¼ cup chopped onion

2 teaspoons curry powder—powerful antioxidants and anti-inflammatory compounds

½ teaspoon salt

¾ cup water

Preparation:

Cook all ingredients, covered, on the stove for approximately 20 minutes, or combine the ingredients in a rice cooker and cook until the rice is slightly al dente.

Coconut Milk: Benefits for Hair

Coconut milk is rich in protein and other nutrients, and this makes it good for healthy hair growth. It is one of the popular and effective kitchen remedies for better hair. Topical application of coconut milk is claimed to boost hair growth and counter dandruff and even hair loss. Regular use of coconut milk and/or coconut oil is also found to reduce the rate of graying. It can make your mane softer and is also used as a hair conditioner.

You can use ready-made coconut milk from supermarkets, but fresh is always best for both culinary and cosmetic purposes. Prepare 2 cups of lukewarm coconut milk and gently massage it onto the scalp. Leave it for at least an hour, before rinsing with lukewarm water. You may use a small amount of herbal shampoo to wash the hair. Repeat this procedure at least once a week for increased results.

ASIAN-STYLE SHRIMP and PINEAPPLE FRIED RICE

<u>Makes 6 Servings</u>

*T*his dish makes for a terrific main course for a casual dinner. There's nothing quite like warm fruit and this recipe is pretty close to the one my mother used to make when entertaining. This version's got a bit of a Hawaiian vibe to it—the mixture of pineapples and shrimp is delicious. The omega-3s in shrimp are good oils for hair health.

Ingredients:

1 (4-pound) pineapple
½ cup julienned red bell pepper—carotenoids
3 scallions, sliced thin—antioxidants
2 teaspoons minced fresh jalapeño pepper, including the seeds, or to taste
1½ tablespoons soy sauce
1½ teaspoons Truvia Baking Blend
1 teaspoon anchovy paste—vitamin A, calcium, potassium, selenium
½ teaspoon turmeric—antiseptic, antibacterial
1 tablespoon water
2 tablespoons vegetable oil
1 pound small shrimp, shelled and deveined—protein
2 garlic cloves, minced—health booster
4 cups cooked whole grain rice
¼ cup finely chopped fresh coriander—essential oils

Preparation:

1 Halve the pineapple lengthwise and cut out the flesh, leaving ½-inch-thick shells (reserve the shells).

2 Remove the core and cut enough of the pineapple into ½-inch pieces to measure 1½ cups, reserving the remaining pineapple for another use. (You can freeze the pineapple core and save it for a blended smoothie. Tons of vitamins in there!)

3 In a bowl, combine the pineapple pieces, the bell pepper, the scallions, and the jalapeño pepper.

4 In a small bowl, whisk together the soy sauce, Truvia Baking Blend, anchovy paste, turmeric, and the water.

5 In a wok or heavy skillet, heat 1 tablespoon of the oil over moderately high heat until it is hot but not smoking; carefully place the shrimp in for 1½ minutes and stir-fry until they are just firm, then transfer them to a bowl.

6 Heat the remaining 1 tablespoon of oil over moderately high heat until it is hot but not smoking and stir fry the garlic for 5 seconds, or until it is golden. Add the rice and stir-fry the mixture for 30 seconds, or until the rice is hot. Add the soy mixture and stir-fry for 1 minute. Add the pineapple mixture and the shrimp and stir-fry the mixture for 1 minute, or until it is hot; then stir in the coriander.

For an exotic flourish, serve the fried rice in the reserved pineapple shells.

Hydrating Honey-Pineapple Facial Mask

You will need fresh pineapple, 3 tablespoons of extra-virgin olive oil, and 1 tablespoon of organic honey. Mash the pineapple, and add in the olive oil and honey until you have created a smooth paste. Spread the paste on your clean face and neck with your fingertips, gently and equally, keeping the eye area clear. Relax and leave the mask on for 15 minutes. Wash it off with lukewarm water, and close out with a splash of cold. Pat your skin dry with a clean towel. Finally, apply a moisturizer; this way you seal your skin to keep the water inside.

BAKED TILAPIA with SPICY TOMATO-PINEAPPLE RELISH

Makes 4 Servings

*F*ish are among the most hydrating foods for hair. Tilapia is an inexpensive freshwater fish with a mild flavor. Because it does not have a strong flavor of its own, it's the perfect fish to use in recipes that call for marinades, herbs, and spice rubs—it tastes like whatever you put on it. Tilapia is high in protein and low in saturated fat and calorie content.

Ingredients:

4 (6-ounce) tilapia fillets—heart-healthy clean protein
¼ teaspoon kosher salt
½ cup crushed pineapple, well-drained—fresh is best—digestive bromelain
2 plum tomatoes, diced
1 teaspoon Tabasco, or more, to taste—zero calories, zero salt, can help with weight loss

Preparation:

1 Preheat the oven to 375°F. Line a baking sheet with aluminum foil and coat the foil with canola oil spray.

2 Place the tilapia fillets on the prepared baking sheet and season them with the salt.

3 In a small bowl, combine the pineapple, tomatoes, and Tabasco. Divide the topping evenly among the tilapia fillets.

4 Bake for 12 to 15 minutes, or until the tilapia flakes easily with a fork.

The combination of pure ingredients in Tabasco helps nudge your metabolism into action. Capsaicin, the compound that gives chile peppers their spicy kick, can create enough heat to raise your body temperature, which helps you burn more calories after a meal by nearly 8 percent. The hotter the Tabasco, the greater the benefit. You'd have to eat it frequently to get a result, but a teaspoon per meal is a great start.

PISTACHIO-CRUSTED HALIBUT
with SPICY YOGURT

Makes 4 Servings

*H*alibut has a slightly sweet yet mild flavor. It's a lean, cold-water fish rich in selenium. Halibut can help keep skin supple and elastic by preventing cellular damage from free radicals. Cold-water fish are a rich source of omega-3s, a form of essential fatty acids that are essential for health but cannot be made by the body. Time to book that fishing trip!

Ingredients: Halibut

4 (1¼-inch thick) pieces skinless halibut fillet—about 6 ounces each

1 cup whole milk—lactic acid, vitamin D

3 tablespoons cornmeal—gluten free; helps lower cholesterol

⅓ cup finely chopped, shelled pistachios—vitamin E

¾ teaspoon iodized salt

¼ teaspoon black pepper

¼ cup extra-virgin olive oil

Spicy Yogurt

1 cup thick Greek yogurt—probiotic protein source

1 cucumber, peeled, seeded, and finely diced—hydration

2 tablespoons chopped fresh dill—antimicrobial and antioxidant actives

1 tablespoon finely chopped onion

1 tablespoon fresh lemon juice

2 teaspoons red pepper flakes—excellent source of beta-carotene

½ teaspoon iodized salt, or to taste

Preparation:

1 Rinse the fish under cool water and pat dry. Place in a glass baking dish, pour all of the milk over it, then chill, fish covered, turning over once, for 30 minutes.

2 Meanwhile, mix the cornmeal and pistachios in a shallow bowl.

3 Remove the fish from the refrigerator, let the excess milk drip off, and then transfer the fish to a plate. Sprinkle all over with salt and pepper, and then dredge in the cornmeal mixture. Once coated, transfer to a clean plate.

4 Heat the oil in a 12-inch heavy skillet over moderately high heat until hot but not smoking, then sauté the fish, turning over once, until golden and just cooked through, 6 to 8 minutes total.

5 While the fish is cooking, stir together all the spicy yogurt ingredients and serve on the side with the fish.

 Sour Cream/Yogurt Mask for Greasy Hair

Depending on the length of hair, massage 1 to 1½ cups of sour cream or plain yogurt into damp hair and let it sit for 15 minutes. Rinse with warm water, followed by cool water, then shampoo hair as you normally would.

CUCUMBER SALAD with PINEAPPLE and JALAPEÑO

Makes 6 to 8 Servings
---

*T*his is a light and refreshing combination with an interesting balance of tastes. I think it is a unique and sophisticated salad in that it is not something you would see on a typical restaurant menu. Cucumber is the ultimate "neutral" veggie that works well with so many other fruits, vegetables, and spices. Pineapple yields bromelain and digestive enzymes, and (with the exception of Truvia for added flavor) this salad is high in water content due to its all-natural ingredients. Hydration is key for hair health. Drink a tall cold glass of water while you make this salad.

Ingredients:

¾ cup Truvia Baking Blend (Truvia is all natural, made from the licorice leaf; when split with their baking blend, it's half the calories of regular sugar)

⅔ cup white vinegar—assists the body with absorption of essential minerals; also great for kitchen cleaning

2 tablespoons water

½ teaspoon iodized salt

1 cup peeled, cored, ⅓-inch diced, fresh pineapple

1 English hothouse cucumber, cut into ⅓-inch pieces

1 carrot, peeled and cut into matchstick-size strips—beta-carotene source

⅓ cup thinly sliced red onion

1 tablespoon minced, seeded jalapeño chile

1 head green leaf lettuce, leaves separated—provitamin A; milder taste than darker greens with full vitamin supply

1 tablespoon toasted sesame seeds

Preparation:

1 Bring the first four ingredients to a boil in a heavy, small saucepan, stirring until the Truvia Baking Blend dissolves. Simmer until reduced to ⅔ cup and a syrupy consistency, about 4 minutes.

2 Transfer the syrup to a large bowl and refrigerate until cold. Add the pineapple to the syrup. Cover and refrigerate for 1 hour.

3 Add the cucumber and next three ingredients to the pineapple mixture; stir to coat. Line the plates with lettuce leaves. Spoon the salad on top of the lettuce. Sprinkle with the sesame seeds and serve.

Pineapple: Superfood for Skin and Hair!

Pineapple is my number-one celebrity secret for blemishes due to its high *sulfur* content—a good thing! Sulfur is a naturally occurring antibacterial agent that lives in connective tissues, nerve cells, skin, hair, and nails—it is one of the most abundant minerals in the body. It's a key element in cell turnover, which can reduce breakouts, blemishes, and acne. Sulfur also helps the body to create longer, stronger hair. Fresh pineapple is also a great source of vitamin C, which fights free radicals. Pineapple's magical enzyme is bromelain, which aids digestion, and is most heavily concentrated in its core. The small woody center that is the pineapple core is tough, and not nearly as sweet as the flesh; however, it contains digestive enzymes that can also be helpful in combating bad breath. Some people take bromelain digestive enzyme supplements after meals to get the healthy effects of eating pineapple.

OYSTER STEW

Makes 4 Servings

*L*ike opera, oysters are an acquired taste, but these lovely, elegant mollusks are high in protein and low in fat and calories. Oysters are a great source of iron, which plays a role in hair health because it helps red blood cells carry oxygen to the hair follicles. Oysters also have omega-3 fatty acids—you need the fat to help build cell membranes in the scalp, which feeds the hair shafts natural oil. Oysters are rich in vitamins A and C. Vitamin A helps produce and protect scalp oils. Vitamin C helps fight hair breakage. The zinc in oysters is an antioxidant that helps guard against free-radical damage. A deficiency in zinc may result in hair loss over time, so it's good to bone up on it proactively and get your RDA (recommended daily allowance). The copper content in oysters helps the body to produce the pigment called melanin, thus contributing to hair color. Any way you slice it (or slurp it), oysters are good for the hair.

Ingredients:

2 (10.75 ounce) cans low-sodium cream of mushroom soup
2 (8-ounce) cans oysters
2 cups milk
16 ounces crimini mushrooms, halved—high in selenium
¼ cup butter
1 teaspoon salt
1 teaspoon ground black pepper
½ teaspoon ground cayenne pepper

Preparation:

Stir together all the ingredients in a saucepan over medium heat; bring to a simmer and cook until hot, about 12 minutes.

Home-Spa Treatments
for Common Hair Challenges

Like people, hair types and hair challenges come in every shade of the rainbow. And typical of the human nature, everyone wants what they don't have. I want Ali Pearlman's phone-cord curly hair, while she dreams of having smooth hair with waves, like mine. Some spend a small fortune to chemically straighten their locks, or hours to manually straighten them with a flat iron, while others go to bed at night with a head full of curlers. Those who have dry hair wish they had just a touch more oil, while those with oily hair wish for the exact opposite . . . you get the idea. Your hair is the byproduct of what you eat; it receives the benefits of healthy eating habits. Protein and enriched foods, such as meat, beans, and omega-3 fatty acids, found in certain fish like salmon, can also promote hair growth. You can also add protein and omega-3 fatty acids to your diet by taking supplements. At the very least, a multivitamin will help provide an environment for your hair to thrive. Following are a few different hair treatments for some of the more common hair challenges. You, and your hair, will likely fit into one of these categories.

 ## Home-Spa Olive Oil Hair Mask for All Hair Types

Inspired by what the Mediterranean beauties have done for centuries, I use olive oil for hair exuberance. Here's how: Mix 2 tablespoons of extra-virgin olive, 1 ripe avocado for adding shine, and 1 tablespoon of mayonnaise. Apply to hair as a mask—no need to massage it in. Cover hair with plastic wrap and leave on for 12 minutes, then shampoo as usual. This helps repair split ends, heals dandruff caused by dry scalp, and makes your hair shiny, silky, and lustrous.

 ## Extra Conditioning Hair Mask

Mix together ½ of a banana, ¼ of an avocado, 1 tablespoon of wheat germ oil, and 1 tablespoon of Greek yogurt. Pierce 1 vitamin E capsule and squeeze it into the mixture. Apply to hair and leave on for 15 minutes. Vitamin E is an antioxidant that helps protect the scalp's natural oils. This mask helps make your hair shiny.

TIP: Keep blow-drying to a minimum. Although the speediest way to dry your locks, blow-drying more than three times a week will damage hair. Towel-dry hair gently and don't twist or wring it out like a sponge. For more targeted drying, aim the blow dryer on a cooler setting directly at the scalp to dry the moisture. If you have thick hair, you may have noticed that a damp scalp can get itchy by the end of the day so you will want to get to the root of it to remove the moisture. Let the rest air dry.

TIP: Harsh shampoos that are filled with chemicals will strip your hair of its natural proteins. If the protein is not replaced, the hair cuticle weakens, which leads to dry, frizzy hair and split ends.

Corn or Honey for Dry Hair and Scalp

Pour 1 tablespoon of cornmeal or cornstarch into an empty saltshaker and sprinkle it onto dry hair and the scalp until you've used it all. After 15 minutes, use a paddle hairbrush to completely brush it out. You can also massage approximately ½ cup of honey into clean, damp hair, let it sit for 20 minutes, then rinse with warm water. Add 1 to 2 tablespoons of olive oil to the honey to loosen it for easier application.

No More Frizz Banana-Cantaloupe-Yogurt Treatment

In a blender, mix together 1 banana, ¼ of cantaloupe, 2 tablespoons of yogurt, and 1 tablespoon of olive oil. Apply the mixture to damp, unwashed hair and comb through all the way. Let it sit for 20 minutes and then rinse it out. Shampoo and condition your hair. Your hair will be smooth and luxurious.

Plump It Up Conditioner for Flat Hair

In the shower, a large washbasin, or the kitchen sink, combine equal parts of warm hair conditioner and Epsom salt. Work the mixture through your hair and leave it on for 20 minutes. This works for flat hair as the salt helps to increase moisture content when mixed with an emulsion base (a conditioner). Rinse out with lukewarm to cold water (to avoid stripping hair).

Caffeine Bath for Super Shiny Dark Hair

Caffeine can intensify your dark locks and make the color rich so they really stand out! Brew a pot of nonflavored coffee or strong black tea. Pour it into a large bowl, and, while it is quite warm, lean over the bowl and soak your hair in it. (Simply swish your hair around in the liquid.) Comb through, cover your head with a plastic shower cap, and let it sit for 20 to 30 minutes while you read a magazine, catch up on e-mail, watch *American Idol* reruns, or what have you. Rinse it out, shampoo, and rinse again with cold water to give it that super shine!

PRO TIP | Turning down the heat while you shower will maximize skin- and hair-moisture retention. To lock in even more humectants (moisture), try placing an Alka Seltzer tab in the corner of the shower floor to help carbonate steam. If your shower is a larger space, you can use two tablets. Try once a month or once a season. After showering, be sure to moisturize when skin is still damp.

TIP: This should be of concern, especially if you wear your hair short: When turning in for the night, remember to remove your earrings before going to bed. You may be comfortable sleeping with your earrings in, and perhaps you wear this "everyday pair" and never remove them at all. But while you sleep on your side, toss and turn, you are actually tugging your earlobes and ever so slightly agitating the pierced hole. This can lead to a stretched piercing site, which over time starts to look more like a thin line than a hole, and after many years can even split entirely, forming a Pac-Man type of appearance.

Home-Spa Lemon Dandruff Treatment

Washing your hair with a mildly acidic product such as lemon juice helps exfoliate the scalp to prevent dandruff. Other home remedies include mixing equal parts of lemon juice and water and soaking your hairbrush in the mixture for 1 hour. This allows for regular scalp treatment.

Bye-Bye Dandruff

Mix together ½ cup of water and ½ cup of white vinegar. Put the mixture directly on your scalp and then start shampooing. Recommended twice a week for flake-free locks!

TIP: Conditioning hair *before* shampooing takes off the "weight" that thick conditioners can leave behind on your hair. Shampooing second also cleans the conditioner off your back and body that you'd be toweling into your skin.

TIP: Eat spinach, Swiss chard, kale, collards, turnips, romaine, and purple cabbage. They contain vitamins A and C, which help your body produce sebum, a natural scalp oil that moisturizes your hair and combats dryness. The leafy greens are best for you when eaten lightly steamed.

Boost Hair Pigment

African American hair needs extra moisture, so a moisturizing shampoo is best. Conditioners are a must and deep conditioning the hair after every shampoo will make hair stronger and avoid breakage. Deep condition for 20 to 30 minutes under a dryer, or for 45 minutes if using only a plastic cap.

Slow Hair Loss

Are you noticing more frequent hair loss? Is your hair thinning? Are too many stray hairs left behind on your pillowcase? A good friend of mine suggested trying a medical-grade chemotherapy shampoo that can stimulate and speed-up growth. She is now healthy (!) and has a full head of beautiful hair. Ask your doctor or pharmacist, and expect to spend quite a bit on this product.

Tea Tree Benefits

Tea tree oil is an antibacterial essential oil that can increase hair radiance, too. Applied to skin it is tingly and can feel bracing and revitalizing. It's marvelous in shampoos and makes the scalp come alive. Everyday oil, dirt, or dry skin cells in need of a sloughing can cause blocked hair follicles, and this can lead to hair loss. Tea tree oil works great for unblocking the hair follicles. Try adding a dime-size amount of tea tree oil to get more effectiveness out of your shampoo and/or conditioner. A small amount of the oil massaged into the scalp, or a shampoo containing 2 percent of the oil, will unclog the follicles and may even stimulate new hair growth. Tea tree oil applied to the scalp is also a stimulating, natural treatment for dandruff.

Eyes That Love You Back

Chapter 2

Looking for eye clarity? Are under-eye bags weighing you down? Can you put an X-marks-the-spot on obvious eye circles? Look no further for eye enlightenment! In this chapter, I will show you how to treat crepey under eye skin, eat the foods that can help improve vision, and give you my inside tips on beauty treatments for youthful-looking eyes. If you want to smooth the skin around the delicate eye area, are besieged with dark circles (which are usually hereditary), or see the onset of crow's-feet and furrows, these recipes and treatments can help. And if there's one thing we can all see eye-to-eye on, it's that a combination of the right nutrients for inner health and the right treatments for outer health add up to gorgeous. So, what types of foods should you eat?

What You Should Know

Fruits and vegetables with vitamin C, like oranges, grapefruit, strawberries, papaya, green peppers, and tomatoes, should be a big part of your life, if they aren't already. Try to eat a rainbow of colors every day. Vitamin C is *numero uno* for eye health.

Vitamin E, found in vegetable oils (safflower and corn oil), almonds, pecans, wheat germ, and sunflower seeds, among other foods, protects eye cells from damage caused by unstable molecules called free radicals, which break down healthy tissue. Beta-carotene is also essential for eye health. Try eating lots of deep orange or yellow fruits and vegetables, such as

41

cantaloupe, mangos, apricots, peaches, sweet potatoes, and carrots.

Dark green leafy vegetables such as broccoli, collard greens, asparagus, kale, and spinach are the primary sources of lutein and zeaxanthin [zea-ZAN-thin], which promote eye health through their ability to filter out UV light. Get keen on greens! Stat! Please understand that if your eyes are healthy, you will likely be squinting and rubbing them less frequently, and since squinting and rubbing, over time, will cause wrinkling, you definitely want to avoid it!

Zinc is also important. Good sources of zinc include beef, lamb, oysters, eggs, shellfish, milk, peanuts, whole grains, and wheat germ. And of course, who could forget those famous omega-3 fatty acids? You will read a lot about them in this book, but, for now, you can zero in on leafy greens, nuts, fish, soy, flaxseed, and vegetable oils like canola to kick-start your Getting Gorgeous plan. In this chapter, these recipes and ingredients yield more benefits than meet the eye. If you can cook and eat them *and* put them on your skin, you are creating a full cycle of inside-out beauty as a whole! Let's kick it off with my celebrity eye-care treatment. Here's an all-natural evening facial for a revitalized face in the morning. It will help you look like you've Z'd for eight hours when all you got was four:

 ## All-Natural Spinach Facial

Blend 1 cup of frozen spinach with ½ cup of coffee grounds and add 1 cup of Greek yogurt. Apply on face and eyes. Lie down and relax for 5 minutes and then wash off.

Moving forward, here are my personal favorites for hydration and health that yield the best results for eye clarity and eye-area youthfulness. The list could go on and on, but that would be source material for my next book!

TOP 5 Hero Foods for Youthful-looking Eyes

Spinach, and other leafy greens—vitamin C promotes eye health internally.

Garlic—it contains healthy, reliable amounts of selenium. Like lycopene, selenium can protect the eyes from disease.

Tomatoes—their concentrated antioxidant lycopene is a key component of eye health.

Avocados—they have more lutein than any other commonly consumed fruit. Lutein protects against macular degeneration and cataracts.

Bananas—their vitamin compounds preserve the membranes that surround your eyes.

SPINACH PIE

Makes 5 to 6 Servings

Declining eyesight as we age is a slice of humble pie. Just when we thought we had the X-ray vision of youth, we start to see things a little more fuzzily. Spinach is a rich source of lutein, a carotenoid, which is known to help protect against cataracts and other age-related macular degeneration. It has the power to reduce dark circles under the eyes due to its high levels of vitamins K and C.

Ingredients:

7 large eggs—protein blast

2 tablespoons milk, or soy milk

3 roasted garlic cloves, crushed

¼ teaspoon lemon pepper

1 dash salt

3 slices cooked bacon, chopped (optional)

1 large flour tortilla—half the calories of a slice of bread

1½ cups any blend shredded cheese

3 cups fresh spinach—antioxidant power

Preparation:

1 Preheat the oven to 365°F.

2 Mix the first six ingredients (eggs, milk, garlic, lemon pepper, salt, and bacon) in a bowl. Set aside.

3 Lay the flour tortilla in a glass pie dish, and press gently.

4 Sprinkle ½ cup of the shredded cheese on the tortilla.

5 Sprinkle the remaining cheese and the spinach onto the tortilla in layers, and press gently.

6 Pour the egg mixture evenly over the spinach, being careful not to pour any outside of the tortilla as this causes it to stick to the dish.

7 Bake in the oven for 35 to 45 minutes. Insert a fork in the center and it should come out clean.

8 Use a sharp knife to cut into pie slices and serve hot. For added flavor, serve with homemade salsa.

CRUNCHY, CHEESY KALE CHIPS

Makes 4 Snack-Size Servings

*K*ale is the oft-neglected leafy green. Many people are not yet familiar with how to cook it, what to eat it with, or even what it looks like. Kale is a form of cabbage, usually green, in which the central leaves do not form a head; they look more like ragged-edge palm leaves, are slightly rubbery to the touch, and are slightly coarse. Kale is high in antioxidants, containing folate, calcium, and other nutrients that support bone health, protect against cognitive decline, and help prevent age-related eye problems. Loaded with calcium and magnesium, too, these Crunchy, Cheesy Kale Chips are the new chip for food-savvy eaters. You'll want to gobble them up by the bowlful and share them with your neighbors! You'll never feel guilty about eating a crunchy zesty snack that's low in fat and good for you. These are my favorite when topped with a little almond butter dressing.

Ingredients:

1 large bunch kale, cleaned and dried, tough stems removed,
  leaves torn to palm-size pieces
⅓ cup extra-virgin olive oil
½ cup finely grated Parmesan cheese

Preparation:

1 Preheat the oven to 450°F.

2 In a large bowl, use your hands to mix the kale and olive oil until the leaves are coated with oil.

3 Spread the kale evenly in one layer on a cookie sheet, then sprinkle with the cheese. Use two sheets if necessary.

4 Bake for 15 minutes, or until crisp. Eat immediately.

HOMEMADE SALSA

Makes 2 to 3 Cups

*T*rying to dream up something light and simple but packed with flavor? Add salsa to your meal. Salsa adds loads of flavor, jazzing up just about any everyday dish. It's also great with a side of blue corn tortilla chips. This salsa recipe is well worth the chopping time.

Ingredients:

4 medium tomatoes, cored, seeds removed, chopped

2 medium cloves garlic, finely minced

2 to 3 tablespoons finely chopped sweet onion

1 to 2 tablespoons minced jalapeño

2 heaping tablespoons finely chopped cilantro

2 tablespoons fresh lime juice—vitamin-C antioxidant power to protect eyes from aging

Preparation:

In a bowl, combine all the ingredients and stir to blend. Cover and refrigerate until serving time.

 Brightening Lime-Turmeric Face Mask

Vitamin C helps fight cellular damage and improve skin's elasticity. It prevents wrinkles and is known to brighten the complexion. Lime juice has a high amount of vitamin C and alpha hydroxy acids (AHA), which are also known to brighten skin. Turmeric powder acts as a disinfectant and is one of my favorite, natural skin-clarifying secrets! Olive oil works here as a natural moisturizer. This mask will brighten your complexion. You'll need:

1½ teaspoons flour

Pinch of turmeric powder

1 teaspoon olive oil

1 teaspoon whole milk

⅛ teaspoon lime juice or juice from a fresh lime

Mix all the ingredients together in a small bowl. Apply to a clean face, and leave on until your skin begins to feel tight, approximately 15 minutes. **Note:** The potency of this mask expires in about 5 days as the natural process of oxidation affects the ingredients upon exposure to the air. Share it with a friend so you don't waste the magic.

ROASTED GARLIC and KALE SOUP

Makes 4 Servings

*T*his recipe is especially rich in lutein/zeaxanthin, vitamin C, vitamin E, folate, and zinc. It also provides fiber, B vitamins, calcium, copper, iron, manganese, potassium, and selenium. If you're going on a date tomorrow, maybe stay off the garlic tonight and save this recipe for another meal!

Ingredients:

1 medium-size bulb of garlic
1 cup uncooked elbow macaroni—healthy starch
1 tablespoon extra-virgin olive oil
1½ cups diced onion
2 tablespoons chopped fresh sage or 2 teaspoons dried sage—antioxidant
  and antimicrobial properties
8 cups washed, drained, and chopped kale—superfood
1½ pounds sweet potato, peeled and cut into bite-size pieces—superfood
8 cups chicken stock
1 tablespoon McCormick chicken base, or 1 to 2 chicken bouillon cubes
  (optional)
2 (8-ounce) cans butter beans, drained and rinsed—fiber; cardiovascular benefits
Salt and pepper, to taste

Preparation:

1 Heat the oven to 425°F.

2 Wrap the garlic bulb in foil and bake for 40 minutes or until soft. Remove from the foil, cool, and remove the cloves from the papery shell. Set the cloves aside.

3 Cook the macaroni according to the directions on the package until al dente. Drain and set aside.

4 In a large, nonstick skillet, heat the olive oil over medium heat. Add the onions and sage and cook until the onion is transparent, stirring occasionally, approximately 5 minutes. Add the kale and continue to stir for another 5 minutes. Add the sweet potatoes, stock, and chicken base. Bring to a boil, reduce the heat, and simmer until the sweet potato is soft, but still firm, approximately 15 minutes. Simultaneously, add the cooked garlic cloves.

5 Add the macaroni and beans to the soup, add salt and pepper, and heat through for 5 minutes. Serve hot.

PEAR, STILTON, and CHICORY SALAD with CHESTNUTS

Makes 3 to 4 Servings

Chicory has disease-fighting phytochemicals and is one of the top vegetable sources of vitamins A, E, and K, fiber, calcium, potassium, pantothenic acid, copper, and folate. It is loaded with beta-carotene and lutein/zeaxanthin. The chicory variety in this recipe is called curly endive, which has a bitter taste, but, when mixed with other neutralizing vegetables, it makes for a rather pleasing taste combination that's fresh, light, and hydrating. Choose a curly endive with firm leaves of a beautiful green color and no spots.

Ingredients:

4 tablespoons extra-virgin olive oil
2 (8-ounce) jars of roasted, skinned chestnuts—high in fiber
Salt and pepper, to taste
2 Asian pears—vitamin C
1 teaspoon grainy mustard—high in selenium
1 tablespoon sherry
1 tablespoon white truffle oil
1½ tablespoons finely chopped shallots—vitamin A; copper
½ head chicory (aka curly endive), torn—6 cups
½ cup pomegranate seeds—antioxidants
3 ounces Stilton cheese, crumbled—good dairy source

Preparation:

1 Heat 2 tablespoons of extra-virgin olive oil in a 10-inch cast-iron skillet over moderately high heat until hot but not smoking, then sauté the chestnuts with salt and pepper to taste, stirring, until just crisp on the outside, about 4 minutes. Remove from the heat.

2 Core the pears, then cut lengthwise into thin slices.

3 Whisk together the mustard, sherry, salt, and pepper in a large metal bowl and add the remaining 2 tablespoons of olive oil and the truffle oil in a slow stream, whisking until emulsified. Add the shallots, whisk another minute.

4 Next, add in the chicory, chestnuts, pears, half of the pomegranate seeds, and Stilton and toss until evenly coated. Top with the remaining half of pomegranate seeds and season with salt and pepper.

CHICORY with BEANS, TOMATOES, and CROUTONS

Makes 5 Servings
---

*H*ere's another well-balanced dish in keeping with our chicory theme—
a hearty and healthy combo with lots of flavor and texture. And it's got
bread, which is always a pleasure to eat.

Ingredients:

2 (¾-ounce) slices French bread, cut into ¾-inch cubes

1 small garlic clove, crushed

½ pound dried navy beans—high in fiber and folate

1 bay leaf

2 cups water

8 cups chopped curly endive—about 1½ pounds—low-cal high fiber; vitamin A
and folic acid

2⅓ cups diced seeded tomatoes

¼ cup minced fresh basil

2 garlic cloves, minced

½ teaspoon salt

¼ teaspoon pepper

2 teaspoons extra-virgin olive oil

Preparation:

1 Preheat the oven to 350°F.

2 Combine the bread cubes and crushed garlic in a large zip-top plastic
bag. Seal the bag, and shake to coat the bread cubes. Arrange the
bread cubes in a single layer on a baking sheet. Bake for 15 minutes
or until toasted.

3 Sort and wash the beans, and place in a large Dutch oven. Cover the
beans with water to 2 inches above beans. Bring the beans to a boil,
and cook for 2 minutes. Remove the beans from the heat; cover and
let stand for 1 hour. Drain.

4 Add the bay leaf and 2 cups of water to the beans in the pan, and bring to a boil. Cover, reduce the heat, and simmer for 1 hour. Discard the bay leaf. Add the curly endive; cover and cook for 10 minutes, stirring occasionally. Stir in the tomato, basil, garlic, salt, and pepper, and cook, uncovered, for 5 minutes. Spoon the bean mixture into a medium bowl. Drizzle with oil, and top with the croutons.

Variation: *Substitute 2½ cups drained canned beans, such as navy, cannellini, or other white beans, for dry beans. Do not soak canned beans.*

Know Your Chicory

Perhaps the only form of chicory you may be familiar with is that found in "New Orleans Coffee," which New Orleans is pretty famous for (that, and Jazz Fest. If you've never been to Jazz Fest, put it on your Bucket List!). Roasted chicory is the secret to New Orleans–style coffee, which has an aroma like coffee but no caffeine. It is bittersweet, rich, earthy, and I find it to be very satisfying. Better known, however, are chicory leaves, which include radicchio, escarole, Belgian endive, curly endive, and frisée. Chicories are closely related to lettuces and are heartier with a bitter edge. But when mixed among other salad ingredients and a wonderful dressing, chicory harmonizes with the other flavors so its bitterness is less apparent.

CARROT-GINGER SOUP

Makes 4 Servings

*C*arrot soup with ginger is a nutritious and low-fat soup recipe with a touch of sweetness and a touch of spice. It warms the soul and stimulates the blood. It is said that eating carrots helps improve eyesight. This has not been scientifically proven but eating carrots certainly can't hurt, and there is some evidence that suggests that eating carrots may help maintain current vision capabilities. Carrots are high in beta-carotene (a pro-vitamin), which converts into vitamin A. Carrot sticks are a terrific on-the-go snack and also make for a delicious ingredient in a fragrant soup.

Ingredients:
½ yellow onion, diced
¼ cup minced fresh ginger
3 tablespoons olive oil
4 cups chopped and peeled carrots (about 1½ pounds)
3 cups vegetable broth—bullion, liquid
1½ cups pulp-free orange juice—vitamin C
Dash nutmeg—good for treating acne internally
Salt and pepper, to taste
Yogurt or sour cream (optional)

Preparation:
1 In a large pot, sauté the onions and ginger in olive oil until soft, about 3 to 5 minutes.
2 Add the carrots and vegetable broth; reduce the heat to medium. Simmer until the carrots are soft, about 40 minutes.
3 Add the orange juice and stir well.
4 Working in small batches and using a food processor or blender, process the soup until it's smooth.
5 Return the soup to the pot or serving bowl and add the nutmeg, salt, and pepper, stirring well. Serve with a dollop of yogurt or sour cream, if desired.

Acne-911 Facial

If you suffer from acne marks, nutmeg can help make your scars less noticeable. Mix some nutmeg powder with honey to make a paste, then apply to the acne marks. Nutmeg can actually help you achieve smoother and healthier skin.

SEARED TUNA with ORANGE, AVOCADO, and CILANTRO SALSA

Makes About 6 Servings

Hero Recipe!

*O*utta sight! *Every single ingredient in this recipe has health and beauty benefits. A great mix of 100 percent good-for-you ingredients for a truly satisfying meal.*

Ingredients: Tuna

1 tablespoon extra-virgin olive oil

1 clove garlic, minced

2 tablespoons lemon juice

4 (4-ounce) tuna steaks—preferably sushi grade—omega-3s

Salsa

⅓ cup minced red onion

2 oranges, peeled with all pith removed, and cubed—vitamin C

1 avocado, peeled, seeded, and cubed—anti-aging

¼ cup chopped cilantro—can help remove metals (mercury) from body

Juice of 1 lime

Himalayan crystal salt and pepper, to taste

Preparation:

1 Blend the olive oil, garlic, and lemon juice in a shallow pan. Add the tuna, turn to coat evenly, cover, and marinate for up to 1 hour.

2 In a medium bowl, blend all the salsa ingredients. Cover and refrigerate for up to 1 hour.

3 Place the steaks in a nonstick skillet over medium-high heat. Cook 2 minutes per side for medium rare (3 to 4 minutes per side for well done). Serve with salsa spooned over the top.

COLLARD GREEN
MASHED POTATOES

Makes 8 Servings

T*his recipe contains one of the great cruciferous veggies that should be better incorporated into all of our diets due to its incredible health prop-erties. The cholesterol-lowering ability of collard greens may be the great-est of all commonly eaten cruciferous vegetables. The key to collard greens' great nutrient value is vitamin K. Vitamin K acts as a direct regulator of our inflammatory response and helps to protect bones from fracture. Foods that are high in vitamin K promote healthy blood clotting, prevent calcification of blood vessels or heart valves, help prevent postmenopausal bone loss, and more. Collard greens help keep us looking young! They are high in fiber and folate and are especially rich in vitamin C, lutein, and zeaxanthin. If you smoke, imbibe alcohol regularly, or are low in your daily intake of fruits and vegetables, your body needs lutein and zeaxanthin, two of the most abundant carotenoids. Researchers speculate that these carotenoids may promote eye health through their ability to filter out UV light and protect the eyes from developing age-related macular degeneration and cataracts. So much good from this edible plant . . . Popeye would be green with envy.*

Ingredients:

2½ pounds russet potatoes, peeled and cut into large chunks—good starch

1 bunch collard greens, washed, stemmed, cut into ½-inch strips— approximately 8 cups—phytonutrient-, folate-rich leafy greens

2 garlic cloves, minced

⅓ cup water

½ cup fat-free half-and-half cream

1 tablespoon butter

Salt and pepper, to taste

Preparation:

1 Place the potatoes in a large pot of cold water, bring to a boil, reduce the heat, and simmer until tender, approximately 20 minutes. Drain and return the potatoes to the pot.

2 Place the collards and garlic in a large saucepan over medium heat with water *just* covering them. Bring to a simmer and steam covered for 10 minutes or until cooked through but still bright green, stirring occasionally to prevent burning. Be careful not to overcook the collard greens. Remove from the heat.

3 Add the remaining ingredients to the potatoes, along with the collards (drained). Mash or whip to the desired consistency. Add more cream if it's too thick.

SUPER SWEET-POTATO CHIPS

Sweet potatoes are high in vitamins B_6, C, and D, iron, potassium, and magnesium, and rich in beta-carotene, an antioxidant that contributes to shiny hair. In the body, beta-carotene converts to vitamin A and triggers the DNA that's in charge of producing new skin cells and shedding old ones.

Ingredients:

1 large sweet potato, peeled and sliced very thinly, crosswise—use a mandoline if you have one

4 tablespoons kosher salt—has no additives, as opposed to table salt

1½ teaspoons garlic powder

2½ teaspoons black pepper

Preparation:

1 Line your microwave's rotating plate with parchment paper that you cut to fit the plate. If your microwave plate doesn't rotate, you will need to turn the chips halfway through the cooking process.

2 Arrange the sweet-potato slices on the prepared plate, and keep them from touching. They will shrink up a lot but you don't want them sticking together on the plate.

3 Sprinkle lightly with salt, garlic powder, and pepper.

4 Cook at 50 percent to 60 percent power for 7 to 10 minutes, but, like ovens, microwaves vary in heat intensity. Keep a close eye on the potatoes once the edges start curling up. Slices will dehydrate and shrink. Cook until you see browned spots and the slices are just golden brown in the middle and fluted around the edges. Keep a close watch on your first batch so you know how to gauge your microwave.

5 Let the potatoes cool completely before eating. Enjoy on the spot, or store in an airtight container, up to 3 days.

Crepey/Crow's-Feet Sweet-Potato Eye Treatment

The enzymes in sweet potatoes help to increase firmness and smooth out wrinkles. So you don't lose nutrients and moisture, bake a sweet potato in parchment paper, then mash and combine with a dab of Vaseline. Apply to the tops of lids and orbitally around the eye. Do this twice a week; you will feel and see benefits in one application.

GARLIC CHICKEN

*M*ore heart-healthy garlic, this time with protein. I order this dish whenever I see it on a menu.

Ingredients:

2 large cloves garlic, crushed

¼ cup extra-virgin olive oil—wrinkle reducer

¼ cup dry breadcrumbs

¼ cup grated Parmesan cheese

4 skinless, boneless chicken breast halves—protein

Preparation:

1 Preheat the oven to 425°F.

2 Warm the garlic and olive oil to blend the flavors.

3 In a separate dish, combine the breadcrumbs and Parmesan cheese. Dip the chicken breasts in the olive oil mixture, then into the breadcrumb mixture. Place in a shallow baking dish.

4 Bake in the preheated oven for 30 to 35 minutes, until the chicken is no longer pink and the juices run clear.

ROASTED TOMATO and CARAMELIZED ONION FARRO SALAD

Makes 2 Servings

*N*ow we move away from garlic and onto . . . onions! Like garlic, onions also have the enzyme alliinase, which is released when an onion is cut or crushed, and it causes your eyes to water; it also gives onions their strong scent and flavor. The onions in this recipe are caramelized, so their pungency is neutralized. Onions are great for their organic sulfur compounds that provide health benefits, including strength and resiliency for hair. Farro is a gluten-free grain that's a great substitute for refined wheat pasta or rice. It has a nutty flavor similar to brown rice. It can be found in the supermarket grains aisle. Lycopene from tomatoes is your major eye benefit here.

Ingredients:

2 cups cherry tomatoes

2 tablespoons extra-virgin olive oil

1½ teaspoons salt

½ teaspoon crushed red chile flakes

1 tablespoon butter

2 medium yellow onions, sliced

2 tablespoons balsamic vinegar

1 cup farro—high in fiber and calcium

¼ cup coarsely chopped parsley

TIP: To prevent tears while chopping onions, try any of the following: 1) use a very sharp knife. The enzymes are released when cells are broken or crushed; using a sharp knife slices through the onion rather than crushing it, and, thus, fewer enzymes are released; 2) chill your onions in the freezer for 10 to 15 minutes before cutting them; or 3) cut the onion under water.

Preparation:

1 Place a rack in the center of the oven and preheat the oven to 375°F. Place the cherry tomatoes on a rimmed baking sheet. Drizzle with 1 tablespoon of olive oil, and sprinkle ¾ teaspoon of salt and the red chile flakes. Bake for 15 minutes, or until some tomatoes have burst and are golden brown and sizzling. Remove from the oven and set aside to cool slightly.

2 Mix 1 tablespoon of olive oil and the butter in a large saucepan over medium heat. Add the sliced onions and toss to coat. Allow the onions to cook down for 5 minutes without stirring. Toss after 5 minutes, then allow to cook without being disturbed for another 5 minutes. Add the remaining ¾ teaspoon of salt and toss. The onions will begin to brown. Remove from the heat momentarily, keep your nose back, and add the balsamic vinegar. Toss to coat all of the onions. Return to the heat and allow the onions to cook down to a very caramelized consistency.

3 Bring 4 cups of water to a boil in a large pot. When the water boils, add a pinch of salt. Add the farro and stir. Cook the farro until it is softened and has a light al dente bite to it, about 15 to 20 minutes. Drain the farro in a strainer, return to the pot, and toss with olive oil. Add the roasted tomatoes, caramelized onions, and chopped parsley. Toss and serve warm.

CARAMELIZED TOMATO BRUSCHETTA

Makes 8 Servings

W*hether you like your tomatoes raw, cooked, caramelized, stewed, or juiced, their center-stage antioxidant, lycopene, may have a role in preventing cancer. Studies are ongoing but this is the current wisdom and I'm on board with it. Lycopene has also been shown to improve the skin's ability to protect itself against harmful UV rays in addition to its benefits to overall eye health.*

Ingredients:

1 slender (8-ounce) baguette
3 tablespoons extra-virgin olive oil—moisturizing
1 pint large cherry tomatoes, halved
About ¼ teaspoon each iodized salt and pepper
¾ cup whole-milk ricotta cheese—calcium
1 cup small fresh basil leaves

Preparation:

1 Heat the grill to medium (350° to 450°F).

2 Cut 16 rounds from the baguette. Set the baguette slices on a tray to carry to the grill and brush all over with about 1 tablespoon of oil.

3 Grill the bread with the lid down, turning once with tongs, until browned, 1 to 3 minutes total. Transfer to a platter.

4 Heat a large cast-iron skillet or other ovenproof frying pan on the cooking grate with the grill lid down until water pops when sprinkled on the skillet, 8 to 10 minutes. Add 1½ tablespoons of oil and spread with a heatproof brush. Pour the tomato halves into the pan, then quickly turn with tongs so that all are cut-side down. Sprinkle with ¼ teaspoon each of salt and pepper. Cook with the grill lid down, without stirring, until the juices evaporate and the tomatoes are blackened on the cut side, 10 to 15 minutes. Gently loosen the tomatoes from the pan with a wide metal spatula as they're done and transfer them to a bowl.

5 Spoon the ricotta into a bowl and drizzle the remaining ½ tablespoon of oil on top. Put the basil in another bowl. Set out the toasts with the tomatoes, ricotta, and basil so people can build their own bruschetta. Season with more salt and pepper, to taste.

PROTEIN NUT SALAD

Hands down, this is the best salad I've ever had—my mom's recipe. Romaine lettuce is a complete protein—it has all eight essential amino acids. Cashews offer another blast of protein and mix deliciously with fruits.

Ingredients: Salad

4 heads romaine lettuce, torn into bite-size pieces—antioxidant power

1 (16-ounce) can unsalted raw cashews

1 large fresh pineapple, cut into small pieces—bromelain

1 cup fresh coconut flakes

2 small (11-ounce) cans mandarin oranges, drained

1 large avocado, chopped in chunks

Dressing

½ cup sugar

½ cup vinegar

1 cup canola or vegetable oil

1 teaspoon poppy seeds

⅓ cup finely chopped white onion

Pinch of dry mustard

Preparation:

Combine the salad ingredients in a large bowl. Add the avocado last to keep it from getting mushy or browning. Set aside. Combine the dressing ingredients in a blender and blend until completely combined. Pour the dressing over the salad ingredients just before serving.

CHICKEN TORTILLA SOUP
(Or HOW to KEEP YOUR TEENAGER HOME for DINNER)

Makes 8 Servings

M̲y auntie used to make this recipe for the family when we had big week-end gatherings and meals together, spending time in Visalia, California, watching the days go by. All the cousins came running when she called out for la cena de sopa.

Ingredients:

2 cloves garlic, crushed

3 tablespoons coconut oil

1 package Nueva Cocina Chipotle Taco seasoning (an all-natural, gluten-, dairy- and soy-free brand)

2 (16-ounce) cartons low sodium chicken broth

1 teaspoon chile powder, to taste—beta-carotene, a form of vitamin A, provides antioxidants

Juice of 1 large lime

2 pounds shredded organic boneless chicken breast—protein

1 (14.5-ounce) can stewed Mexican tomatoes—tomatillos are high in potassium and, when ripe, can be yellow, red, green, or purple

1 (15-ounce) can diced chile peppers—mild or hot, depending on preference

Salt, to taste, approximately ½ teaspoon

1 package frozen baby white corn—contains compounds zeaxanthin and lutein for eye health

1 large avocado, as topping

Shredded cheddar cheese, as topping

Chopped scallions, as topping

4 flour or corn tortillas, sliced into strips and baked until crisp (5 minutes at 350°F), coated with olive oil, salt, and pepper.

Preparation:

1 In a large pot, sauté the garlic in coconut oil, then add the seasoning packet and sauté for another few minutes. Next, add 2 cups of chicken broth and let simmer for 5 to 7 minutes. Add the chile powder after simmering. Stir. Add the lime juice.

2 While sautéing, boil the chicken in the remaining broth until cooked almost through (time will vary depending on the thickness of the chicken). Skim the froth from the top during cooking. When the chicken is cooked, remove it from the broth and let it cool until you can shred it using a fork. Shred the chicken into medium-size pieces.

3 Add the garlic mixture to the broth in the pot. Add the tomatoes, chile peppers, salt, corn, and shredded chicken. Simmer for an hour more, then transfer to serving bowls. Serve with chopped avocado, cheddar cheese, and scallions as toppings, and sliced tortillas for dipping.

PAPAYA AVOCADO SALAD

Makes 4 Servings

Add tropical flare to your salad and get the benefits of enhanced digestion, too. Papaya offers the only food source of papain, an anti-inflammatory enzyme that breaks down proteins. Papayas also have 33 percent more vitamin C than oranges. When buying ripe papayas, feel for firm (not hard) fruit. It should have a yellowish rind that has no spots or bruises.

Ingredients:

4 ripe papayas, divided

2 small avocados, diced (1 cup)

⅓ cup chopped raw cashews

¼ cup coarsely chopped fresh mint

3 tablespoons fresh lime juice

1 medium shallot, finely chopped (about 2 tablespoons)

Salt and pepper, to taste

1 cup coarsely chopped, packed arugula

Preparation:

1 Halve 2 papayas and scoop out the seeds. Set the halves aside. Peel the remaining 2 papayas with a vegetable peeler, then halve and scoop out the seeds. Cut the peeled papaya halves into ½-inch dice, and place in a medium bowl.

2 Add the avocados, cashews, mint, lime juice, and shallot to the diced papayas in the bowl, and toss to combine. Season with salt and pepper. Fold in the arugula. Fill the papaya halves with salad, and serve immediately.

JAZZY OATMEAL-BANANA COOKIES

Makes 30 Medium-Size Cookies

O *atmeal often goes hand in hand with cinnamon, and this recipe is no different. However, with these delicious cookies you also get brain-boosting and body-con ingredients. The potassium in bananas provides fuel and helps reduce dehydration, cramping, and fatigue. Cinnamon contains potent antibacterial properties. One of my grandma's swear-by natural acne cures is to apply a mixture of honey and cinnamon powder. "Sweetheart, it's an effective remedy from many moons ago," she used to say when I was in my twenties and struggling with cystic acne. "Trust Va-Va, your skin will clear and you'll feel jazzy again," is what my Portuguese grandmother said.* In this recipe, the banana and oatmeal combination has a slightly "expansive" effect, making you feel satisfied and full more quickly than other flatter cookies may.*

*****P.S.** *Reducing irritation is vital to clearing acne, so never scrub it. Anything that rubs, scratches, or scrubs the skin can cause irritation, so stay very gentle with your towel and avoid washcloths on acne.*

Ingredients:

3 cups rolled oats, old-fashioned
  or instant
1 teaspoon Truvia Baking Blend
½ teaspoon iodized salt
¼ teaspoon baking soda
2 dashes cinnamon

¼ cup cacao powder—the darker,
  the better
3 medium-ripe bananas—moisturizing
¼ cup applesauce
2 tablespoons grapeseed oil
  —moisturizing

Preparation:

1 Preheat the oven to 350°F.

2 Lightly grease two baking sheets.

3 In a large bowl, whisk together the oats, Truvia Baking Blend, salt, baking soda, cinnamon, and cacao. Set aside.

4 In a medium bowl, mash the bananas to a creamy consistency using the back of a fork or a potato masher. Blend in the applesauce and grapeseed oil until thoroughly combined.

5 Mix the liquid ingredients into the dry ingredients.

6 Roll into small balls and drop onto the prepared baking sheets. Flatten the balls slightly with the palm of your hand.

7 Bake for 15 minutes or until crispy and slightly firm. Remove from the baking sheet once the cookies have cooled.

 ## Va-Va's Oatmeal Acne Facial

Mix together ½ cup of oatmeal, 2 teaspoons of honey, ½ teaspoon cinnamon, and ¼ cup of baking soda. Apply and leave on for 15 minutes, Sweetheart.

 ## Almond Oatmeal–Exfoliating Mask

Exfoliating removes the surface layer of dead cells, allowing your freshest skin to shine through. Depending on a few factors such as age and the climate in which you live, most women should exfoliate 1 to 2 times weekly and men should exfoliate 2 to 3 times weekly. You'll need:

½ cup almond milk
2 tablespoons rolled oats
2 tablespoons avocado
½ cup almonds

Add the ingredients to a blender in the order listed and secure the lid. Blend until pasty (approximately 30 seconds) and press "Pulse" to stop the cycle. This recipe yields enough for two masks. You can store any extra in the fridge and use the next day, or do your mask with a pal.

 ## Baking Soda Facial

Believe it or not, baking soda is instrumental in acne control (but not for sensitive skin). For clearing acne with baking soda you have to prepare a thick paste by mixing baking soda powder with water. Apply it over the acne and wait for 15 minutes. Do not rub or circle roughly into skin as this can irritate the epidermis. Wash with cold water. In the treatment, the baking soda acts as an exfoliator and removes the dead skin cells and excess oil that are responsible for causing acne. To balance the pH, follow this treatment with diluted lemon juice or apple cider vinegar blotted gently on the face with a cotton ball, or dab with a Q-tip cotton swab for targeted application.

BLUEBERRY and BANANA COTTAGE CHEESE PARFAIT

Makes 1 Serving

An easy-to-assemble snack that's quick, delicious, nutritious, and bursting with flavor. These tangy sweet berries are wild with flavors that compliment a multitude of desserts, jellies, and jams—and cosmetic products, too. Paired with creamy and satisfying cottage cheese, this protein/antioxidant rich combo is a one-two punch against aging. Blueberries also have a high water content, which makes them great for hydration. And since dehydration usually shows first in our face—around the eyes—blueberries are another go-to food for eye-area improvement. I do, however, try to avoid eating them while drinking my morning coffee, as the two in combination are abrasive on teeth and may cause staining. Enjoy your blueberry parfait with a hot cup of antioxidant-rich green tea instead.

Ingredients:

½ cup cottage cheese
½ cup frozen or fresh blueberries—low-cal superfood
½ cup sliced banana
½ tablespoon toasted, ground, organic flaxseeds—omega-3s
2 tablespoons cinnamon granola
Maple syrup, to taste—zinc

Preparation:

1 Layer cottage cheese, blueberries, and bananas in a tall ice cream glass or parfait cup. One layer of cottage cheese followed by one layer of blueberries, then bananas and so forth.

2 Sprinkle the toasted flaxseeds and granola on top.

3 Drizzle maple syrup over all.

4 Garnish with extra blueberries on top.

Are You Flax-able?

Flax is a fantastic superfood high in omega-3 fatty acids. Ground flaxseed can be tossed into yogurt, cereal, smoothies, muffins, granola—just about any baked good can benefit from their slightly sweet, nutty taste. Flaxseeds are difficult to digest so they should be ground into meal. If you're ready to commit, these flax babies can do a world of good.

 Banana Eye Mask Facial

This might be the easiest facial in the world (!) and requires but two ingredients: a banana and Vaseline. The peel and fruit of the banana contain firming fibers and anti-inflammatory extracts. This eye pack treatment helps reduce loose skin around the eyes, dark circles, crepey skin, wrinkles, lines, and swelling. Too good to be true? Of course not! Try this: Chill the jar of Vaseline in the refrigerator overnight. Take the banana out of the peel and run a large spoon from the top of the peel to the bottom until you strip all the internal fibers. The fibers are actually those white stringy strips that can be found between the banana and the inside of the peel itself. In a metal bowl, mix the banana and the fibers with a quarter-size amount of the cold Vaseline. Apply the mixture to your eyelids and on the top of your eyebrows. Allow it to set for five minutes and then gently wipe it off with a soft tissue. Notice the wide-awake look in your gorgeous peepers? You are now ready for makeup application, but take care to remove all the excess Vaseline—an icy washcloth works best.

Here's another trick you can do with the banana fruit: Mash the banana gently in a small bowl and add a quarter-size amount of Vaseline. Place the mixture in the freezer for five minutes and then apply it under your eyes for five minutes. Gently tissue off with a makeup remover wipe or icy washcloth.

PRO TIP

If you have oily skin, you also have oily eyelids—so you can use a cheek stain on your eyelids for a dreamy effect that smears in just the right way. Oily eyelids look healthy on the beach, dewy in humid weather, and fashion-magazine worthy when coupled with cheek stain to pump up your "eye drama." Embrace your attributes and let them shine forth!

GO-FOR-GORGEOUS GRANOLA

Makes 10 Servings

This is a nutty recipe, so if you have allergies simply skip it and move onto the next. Many granolas are made up of oats, honey, puffed rice, and sugar, but I add nuts for amplified health benefits that move away from the carbs a bit and closer to the proteins.

Ingredients:

2 lemons, zested

½ lemon, juiced

1½ oranges, zested and juiced

⅓ cup extra-virgin olive oil

½ cup pure maple syrup (or ¼ cup maple and ¼ cup honey)

2 egg whites

1 tablespoon vanilla extract—antioxidant properties

4 cups organic rolled oats

1 cup raw cashews—protein and healthy fats

½ cup raw sunflower seeds—cardiovascular benefits

¼ cup raw sesame seeds

½ cup unsweetened dried coconut

¼ cup ground flaxseed

¼ cup wheat germ

1 cup dried fruit—preferably apricots, bananas, cranberries, and papaya

Preparation:

1 Heat the oven to 350°F. Stir the zest, juice, extra-virgin olive oil, syrup, egg whites, and vanilla together in a medium-size bowl.

2 In a large bowl mix the oats, ½ of the nuts, ½ of the sunflower seeds, all the sesame seeds, and the coconut. Stir in the syrup mixture. Spread thinly on two cookie sheets covered in parchment paper or tinfoil for easy cleanup.

3 Bake for 15 minutes, then stir the granola on the trays with a wooden spoon. Continue to bake for 7 minutes or until golden brown. Remove and cool.

4 Stir in the remaining nuts, flaxseed, wheat germ, and dried fruit. When completely cooled, store in airtight containers and enjoy for up to a month, or keep in the freezer for up to 6 months.

) Oatmeal-Parsley-Spinach Reparative Facial

Oatmeal, parsley, and spinach—kitchen staples you likely already have—combine to make a simple healing facial mask for most skin types. Parsley is a natural cleanser full of vitamins and minerals that can stimulate circulation and help release impurities. Sure, it tastes bitter, but when combined with spinach and oatmeal, parsley creates a scrub that leaves your skin looking *sweet*.

In a small bowl, mix ½ cup of finely ground oatmeal with ½ cup of fresh parsley and ½ cup of spinach to make a smooth paste. (If your supermarket does not carry finely ground oatmeal, use a coffee grinder to grind up your oatmeal at home.) As the parsley and spinach are stirred around and agitated in the bowl, they will release water to create a binder. Work the mixture into a paste and apply to a clean face. You may look like you got stuck in a salad wind tunnel, and bits of greenery may be falling off your mug; so if you can relax with a magazine that would be ideal. Leave the paste on for 20 to 30 minutes. Rinse off using lukewarm to cool water. You should see a noticeable improvement in your complexion.

WATERMELON SALSA

Makes 4 Servings

*T*his is a delicious side salad or salsa topping for fish, meat, or chicken. *All natural and loaded with vitamins, it's incredibly good for you. The high-water content and antioxidant lycopene in watermelon are keys for eye health.*

Ingredients:

3 cups diced watermelon
1 large mango, diced small
½ large onion, diced small
2 jalapeño peppers, seeded, rinsed, and diced extra fine
Juice of 2 small limes
1 teaspoon white balsamic vinegar, or distilled white vinegar
1 teaspoon California ground chile (mild)
½ teaspoon cumin
½ bunch cilantro, stems removed, chopped
Salt, to taste

Preparation:

Toss together the watermelon, mango, onion, and jalapeños. Add the lime juice, white balsamic (or distilled) vinegar, ground chile, and cumin. Toss again. Add the chopped cilantro and toss again, and salt, to taste. Note: the salt may cause the melons to expel too much juice; if the salsa gets too watery, drain off the excess before serving.

It is said that 80 to 90 percent of all communication is nonverbal. That means the body, smile, and eyes are doing a lot of the talking. Now that you've learned from this chapter what foods and home-spa treatments you can enjoy and experiment with for improved eye health and eye-area youthfulness, you're set to turn back on your flirty gaze! Remember, we can rarely hide our emotions with our eyes. So if you feel good, everyone will see it, and react accordingly, too.

Of course, feeling good is a top priority, but looking good is also high up on the list, no? In the following chapter we delve into recipes, spa treatments, and information that will feed your face to fabulous.

Caring for the Eyes: Common Challenges

Many of us grapple with eye-area challenges, be it wrinkles, fatty deposits, puffiness, or dark circles. Since there is only so much that cosmetic concealers can do, we must also fight to maintain—or not further age—a youthful eye-area appearance. Let's go over a few of the basics.

1) **Don't smoke.** Smoking and exposure to UV rays both weaken collagen and cause premature wrinkling and sagging.

2) **Use sunscreen.** Apply sunscreen around the eye area; be careful not to get too close to the lash line. Many sunscreen brands now sell SPF (sun protection factor) eye powder that comes with a tiny brush for delicate application. Color Science has a great one that I recommend.

3) **Moisturize.** Dryness is bad for the eye area. Apply an eye cream nightly. You don't need to spend a lot; most drugstore moisturizers will provide the hydration you need. I also provide you with home-spa treatments for moisture in this chapter.

4) **Wear sunglasses.** You should always wear sunglasses in bright sunlight for protection of the delicate eyelid skin as well as your retinas. They are also helpful for reducing squinting. Cheap (street-vendor or dollar store) sunglasses often don't have the same UV protection that reliable name-brand sunglasses do.

Nothing to Crow About

Squinting causes wrinkles known as crow's feet. Many people squint without even realizing it. This "motion wrinkle" tends to be prevalent in people who are nearsighted; that is, they tend to squint to see objects or read signs in the distance. If you are squinting a lot, it may mean that you need glasses, so please have your vision checked. Or perhaps you just need to be more proactive about remembering to bring—and wear—your sunglasses whenever it's sunny out!

Our Aging Eyelids

The eyelids are often the first area of the face to show the signs of aging. In fact, I know a thirty-year-old woman who had her eyes "done," and truth is, she needed it. She's a marathon runner who trains year-round in every kind of weather. She attributed the sagging of her upper eyelids to the constant physical pressure of running and bouncing up and down. There's a good reason why they make exercise bras, but what can they do for the face? she used to say. The skin of the eyelids is half as thin as the rest of the face and has half the density of naturally moisturizing glands. It is delicate! Plus we blink three thousand times a day, so you can be sure those eyelids are working hard. Add to that smiling, crying, rubbing the eyes, and putting in contact lenses, and you have a recipe for easily traumatized, aged skin. Let's fight the battle!

TIP: To subdue crow's feet or a cakey look around the eyes, lightly dot eye cream on *after* applying concealer, and wear *wraparound* UVA/UVB sunglasses for total coverage of the delicate eye area, essential for staving off wrinkles.

Another term for those motion wrinkles is laugh lines, which, as unfair as it seems, are born of—you guessed it—a lifetime of flexing the muscles in the face while laughing and smiling. Keep smiling, my friend, just do it with more SPF!

An Eye for an Eye: Dark Circles

If you are besieged with circles under your eyes, you can take revenge against those dark shadows. For starters, you probably could steal a few more hours of sleep, but the cause actually might be something you've inherited. On a fundamental level, dark circles are created by a loss of volume in the area around the eye. The less fleshy the padding, the more the orbital bone becomes pronounced, creating a hollow trough that shows up as a dark circle; that's technically called a tear trough. The eye is a very delicate organ. For its protection it is surrounded by a cushion of fat. (The right fats are good!) As we get older that fat tends to protrude, sometimes even at a young age. Add that bulge that casts a shadow to a deepened tear trough and you get dark circles. The sun and ceiling lights—light that shines from above us—cast light downward, making angles and shadows along the way. So the shadow they cast under eye-area fat pads are almost impossible to camouflage, even with concealer. You can't remove a shadow unless you hold a light under your chin. Although there are many reasons behind dark circles, such as tiredness and heredity, one of the root causes can be poor circulation. In cases where this is a problem, increasing your intake of vitamins K and C can alleviate them by helping to boost circulation and strengthening capillary walls.

It's very rare, but possible, that dark circles can be caused by irregular skin pigmentation. It's easy to mistake dark circles, which come from vascular problems, with those that come from pigmentation problems. Excessively bulging eyes and/or eyelids also can be an early sign of a condition in that butterfly-shaped neck gland—the master gland of metabolism—the thyroid.

 ## Dark Circles Eye Treatment

Yellow cumin powder mixed with a thick moisturizer is a great natural concealer. It also fights the signs of aging and, as an added benefit, lightly pigments the skin even after you remove it.

If cumin doesn't help, try an under-eye concealer or moisturizer that includes 2 to 5 percent vitamin K. There is anecdotal evidence that vitamin K helps remove dark circles by stabilizing the tiny blood vessels that are in the eyelids and reducing microbleeds and blood-caused pigmentation. Bilberry and vitamin B_3 are also good. Google anything that may interest you in this area and have fun educating yourself.

Apply cucumber juice to eyes with cotton balls and place one cold tea bag on each eye. Use caffeinated teas bags, not herbal, as the caffeine vasoconstricts, which is what you want.

Chomping on crushed ice throughout the day can aid lymphatic drainage and help prevent dark circles around your eyes. This is a long-term fix. Or, press an ice cube up against the roof of mouth to help dissipate the liquid pools in the under-eye bags. Ice externally and internally helps aid the body to reduce inflammation. I teach my celebrity clients this trick to look well rested.

Tired of Looking So Tired?

Baggy, puffy skin under the eyes is usually caused by water buildup under the eyes. The thinnest skin on the face is around the eyes, so it's the area that's most influenced by the in-and-out flow of fluids. Water always travels from areas in the body where there's low salt concentration to tissues where there's more salt. Therefore, a meal high in sodium, or a night of crying while watching your favorite television drama or a sad movie, can cause morning-after puffiness.

TIP: Try changing your sleep position—it may be contributing to under-eye bags. If you're a side sleeper, you may notice a heavier bag on the side you sleep on. No thanks to gravity, sleeping on your side or stomach can direct fluids under your eyes. Try sleeping on your back, or add a thin extra pillow under your head. Some tout the benefit of a silk pillowcase, but I think they can cause acne. At a minimum, a high thread-count cotton pillowcase will work overnight toward skin clarity. **FYI:** Fabric softener can leave a waxy residue on pillowcases, which may aggravate acne. If you have acne anywhere on your body, you should be using a free-and-clear type of laundry detergent without dyes, perfumes, and abrasive chemicals.

Seasonal allergies can also cause puffy eyes. Treat hay fever, if that's the problem. There are nonsedating, over-the-counter allergy medications that may help. Talk with your specialist about how to treat it, and start early in the season to get ahead of the allergy symptoms. You can also try irrigating the nasal cavity with a neti pot—a device that looks like a small teapot—to help relieve fluid buildup caused by allergies, sinus congestion, or a cold.

Aside from the discomfort allergies cause, it's also important to get allergies under control so you stop rubbing your eyes. If you have itchy, watery, burning, sensitive eyes due to pet or seasonal allergies, the common way you soothe them is by rubbing, right? Sometimes we can rub our eyes so hard just to get an ounce of relief that what we are doing, in effect, is disrupting not only the natural pH in the eyes, but aggravating the delicate skin around the eyes.

Don't Take the Red Eye

Lack of sleep, time zone changes, and environment could be causing your bloodshot eyes. If the blood vessels in your eyes are prominent (if your eyes are constantly red), this could be due to sun, wind, dust, smog, and/or pollen, or a deeper cause. If your eyes sting, itch along the lash line, or are itchy in general, you can control a lot of the redness and discomfort by using saline drops, which will moisturize. (Remember, water goes where the salt is.) But you should consult your professional about your condition. Also know that too many eye drops, or the wrong combination of them can sometimes be a culprit here, too. For optimal function and comfort, you want to maintain homeostasis in the eyes, just as you do in the rest of your body.

Get Pretty, not Puffy

If you have puffy eyes, like I do, you need to hyperhydrate. To combat those telltale puffy eyes of mine, I start by using a gel moisturizer to treat the eye area. Then I take a large spoon and run it under hot water to warm it, and gently place the convex side under eye "bags" for a few seconds. Then I alternate with super cold water. This helps depuff quickly while you target the one area. Adding old coffee grounds to the gel moisturizer helps speed up the process. A dab of Preparation H to puffiness once in a while does the trick, too.

TIP: If you have flakiness around the eye area due to bitter cold weather, try gently dabbing Aquaphor or Vaseline at night to dry patches. Do not get too close to the lash line when applying.

TIP: To combat puffy eyes, apply your favorite eye cream with a visible thick coat on your entire orbital eye area. Top with a thin layer of Vaseline. Throughout the night your eyes will be constantly conditioned and moisturized. Puffy eyes need hydration to help depuff.

Time to Feed Your Face

Chapter 3

On the quest for flawless, lit-from-within skin, I have found that there are a myriad of things you need to do if you want to achieve your skin-care goals. Advertisements claim fountain of youth solutions and encourage us to buy, and doctors offer them and encourage us to spend—they don't call it a "pretty penny" for nothing. The untarnished truth? What's on your plate matters most of all. Eating the right kinds of high-performance foods will power your skin and your body. Here's a quiz: which will make you feel healthier, brighter, and glowy—a croissant or a berry parfait? What you eat has *everything* to do with the condition of your complexion. People have different skin types that can be divided into five categories: oily skin, dry skin, normal skin, sensitive skin, and combination skin, which is the most common. Having combination skin means that your face most likely has an oily zone that includes your forehead, nose, and chin, while the rest of your skin has normal to dry patches. When buying a face cleanser, avoid the three S's: soaps, scrubbers, and scents. Look for the words "gentle," "for dry, sensitive skin," and "glycerin," a moisturizing ingredient often included in non-overdrying cleansers.

If you are in your twenties, you may be addressing pimples and clogged pores and will want to be thinking about your skin care in terms of proactive prevention. Regarding what's causing pimples, it could be hormonal, or the choice of foods you are putting into your body. I recommend a good facial every six weeks. My quickie home-remedy fix for blemishes:

The iodine in basic Visine helps shrink pimples and remove redness. Also, rice or almond flower are pressed- and loose-powder alternatives to standard cosmetic powders—without the clogging. For all-day oil control, blot face with rice papers, tissue paper, or sanitary toilet seat covers!

To further fight breakouts, get in touch with your inner chef. You may not be cooking for yourself yet, but that doesn't mean you can't start to cook your way to gorgeous. You should also be proactive about protecting your face *and* neck from too much sun. The rays you are catching now will reveal themselves as brown spots and wrinkled skin fifteen years from now. Just because a suntan fades doesn't mean the damage it does fades with it. Repeated sun exposure depletes the body's antioxidant content, allowing in free radicals that attack cellular lipids, proteins, and even DNA. In laywoman's terms, those spring break days of roasting in the sun are gone, baby, gone. But if you do get burned, postsunburn, chill your aloe vera for an hour before applying. The coolness will help the sensation of burning and help calm redness and inflammation. In your day-to-day activities, you should be wearing sunscreen when the sun is out. There are plenty of nongreasy SPF formulations available today, but, if sunblock makes you feel greasy, add a pinch of cornstarch to your daily SPF to help mattify your skin while you protect it.

Freckles and Melanin

Freckles are the result of a lot of melanin bunched together. But what is melanin? At the base of your epidermis are melanocytes, cells that produce a pigment—that's melanin, and everyone has the same number of melanocytes. The amount of melanin that the cells produce determines the shade of your skin. African Americans and those with darker skin are less prone to melanoma because their skin naturally produces more melanin, and melanin not only creates color but also offers protection from UV exposure. You get a suntan (or sunburn) when your body hyperproduces melanin in order to protect you from harmful sun rays. Those innocent freckles are trying to protect you as minishields. Skin protection for the entire body is especially important in regions that are less frequently exposed to the sun, as that skin is prone to burning faster.

If you are in your thirties, you are probably beginning to notice subtle fine lines or enlarged pores from old acne scars. You may also be noticing that scratches or tiny pimples and scabs on your face don't disappear as quickly as they used to. You're probably still eating everything you crave and your metabolism is working for you just fine ... but wait ... it does slow down, and you end up having to exercise a lot harder to burn off the same amount of calories and fat. You may also still be suntanning, that is, lying on the beach baking in the rays. By the time you're in your thirties, chronic sun damage can start to take hold, which can lead to precancerous and cancerous lesions. You'd be dismayed to learn how common it is for folks in their thirties who discover suspect moles on their skin ... please use caution under the sun! It will catch up with you.

If you are in your forties, don't worry about what you didn't do correctly in your twenties and thirties. You can still work on anti-aging and regain some traction. Eating lots of fresh fruit and vegetables is the way to preventing signs of aging. Essential vitamins and minerals in fresh fruit and veggies work on skin health and elasticity, so make sure you get your 5 to 8 servings of fresh fruit and veggies every day. Also, the time is upon you to get corrective about décolleté brown spots and skin discoloration, wrinkles, subtle under eye circles, and/or eye-area puffiness. You may also have started to notice a loss in skin smoothness and increased freckling. This chapter will address those concerns, too.

In your fifties, dynamic lines, skin luminance, skin brightening and clarity, evenness of skin tone, overall texture, and sagging are likely to be focal issues. Smart eating habits can help with all of these challenges, and taking care of your skin is the difference between healthy skin and less wrinkles. Sticking to a simple skin-care regime every day can make a big difference in how old you look and slow down other signs of aging. Remember, what you put into and on your body shows on the outside, and high performance foods will give your skin more of a high performance appearance.

In your golden sixties, jowls become prominent and nagging. This is a tough area to treat as it is due to age-related loss of collagen/elastin, structural proteins that are hard to replace naturally. You can, however, stick with age-defying, lightening, brightening foods, and treatments and serums for deep repair. You need calcium, concealers, and clarifiers, too. You need great creams and treatments that slow the loss of water and keep the skin supple. Fish, prunes, guava, and blueberries can help.

TIP: My best-kept celebrity secret is using Arnica gel 4 percent for face or body bruising. This is especially useful if you get any type of facial Botox or filler. You can also take Arnica Montana in pill form, for up to a week before injectables. No prescription required.

And my universal, all-for-one and one-for-all desert island recommendations: 1) always wear a high level SPF that has anti-aging properties, and 2) take a multi-omega and flax liquid gel. Stat!

Beautiful, sexy, age-appropriate skin is about long-term choices. If I explained to you that you could eat certain foods that taste great, and, in effect, stimulate cell rejuvenation, would you eat them? (Here's the other part of the quiz.) How about if you were introduced to a host of ingredients and superfoods that not only cut calories and trans fats but actually boost your skin health—would you be open to adding those to your diet? Savvy folks are changing their eating habits and how they nourish their bodies. Food for thought: Skin is the largest organ of the human body weighing more than the human brain. Since over 90 percent of all skin problems start from within, you can believe that what you ingest affects the way you look, and what you eat and put in and on your body therefore affects the way you live. Do the people you know who have gorgeous skin eat Little Debbies and Wonder Bread? Perhaps there's a bigger-picture reason why these factory-made subfoods have disappeared!

TOP 5 Hero Foods for Overall Skin Health

Water—always keep skin hydrated with an atomizer. Continuously misting the skin will help lock in moisture to allow the skin to rebalance itself. This is especially important during air travel.

Polyphenols—free-radical fighters like pomegranates, deep-colored grape juices, and acai berries; the deep color is a polyphenol indicator.

Avocados—omega-3s are needed for healthy glowing skin.

Pink grapefruits—healthy skin-balancing acidity and pink-red hue from lycopene—a carotenoid that may help to keep your skin smooth. Grapefruit balances well with savory dishes.

Leafy greens—they contain beta-carotene, a form of vitamin A, essential for growth and repair of the body's tissues, including skin.

SPF 30+ (sorry, couldn't resist)—it's the easiest way to ward off wrinkles and unsightly sunspots.

POMEGRANATE CHICKEN

<u>Makes 2 Servings</u>

This is another savory/sweet combo that I like and recommend. The pomegranates really play center stage in this dish of very-good-for-you ingredients.

Ingredients:

1 pomegranate

1 pound boneless, skinless, chicken breast halves

1 teaspoon fresh thyme

½ teaspoon salt

½ teaspoon pepper

2 tablespoons red palm oil

1 medium-size onion

2 cloves garlic

½ cup chicken broth

¼ cup orange juice

1 tablespoon grainy mustard

1 teaspoon cornstarch

Preparation:

1 Seed the entire pomegranate, and set aside.

2 Rub the chicken breasts with thyme, salt, and pepper.

3 In a large skillet, heat the red palm oil over medium heat until hot. Add the chicken and cook for 10 minutes, turning once. Remove the chicken.

4 Add the onion and garlic to the skillet. Cook for 5 to 7 minutes until the onion is golden.

5 Return the chicken to the skillet.

6 In a small bowl, whisk the broth, orange juice, mustard, and cornstarch. Add to the skillet. Cook for 1 to 2 minutes until thick.

SKIN-BALANCING CHICKEN STRIPS

Makes 2 Servings

This delicious dish is rich in antioxidants and vitamins A, C, and E, which are beneficial to every skin type, especially those with aging skin. It's a go-to nutritious and tasty meal for any household.

Ingredients:

2 mangoes, peeled, seeded, and chopped

3 tablespoons honey

¼ cup lime juice

¼ cup oil

3 tablespoons low-sodium soy sauce

½ cup fresh pomegranate juice—antioxidants

6 boneless, skinless chicken breasts, halved—protein powerhouse

Preparation:

1 Place the mangoes, honey, and lime juice in a blender; cover and blend until smooth. Place the mango mixture in a covered bowl in the refrigerator.

2 Mix the oil, soy sauce, and pomegranate juice in a small bowl to make a marinade.

3 Cut the chicken into strips and place in a glass pan. Pour the marinade over the chicken. Cover and marinate for 4 hours.

4 Set the oven to broil. Thread the chicken onto metal skewers and cook for 8 to 10 minutes, turning once, until done. Serve with the mango sauce.

GRAPE JELLY

Makes 20 Servings

Grape jelly is a classic that can be enjoyed with everything from whole-grain toast and peanut butter to red apples and cheese. When you make it from scratch, the satisfaction factor is even higher, and the sugar content is lower.

Ingredients:

4 cups 100 percent dark grape juice

1 tablespoon powdered pectin (a thickener)

2 cups Truvia Baking Blend

Preparation:

Bring the juice to a simmer over medium-high in a large saucepan. Whisk in the pectin and cook, whisking occasionally, for 3 minutes. Lower the heat to medium-low; add the Truvia Baking Blend, whisking until dissolved, about 5 minutes. Let the mixture cool slightly before pouring into jars and refrigerating.

SPICED GRAPE BUTTER

Makes About 4 Cups

This is a rustic spread that tastes amazing on toast or tea cookies. It's also wonderful served with a hearty loaf of country bread, accompanied by a warm cup of tea. "Purple fairy paste" is what my friend calls it to sell it to her kids, and since kids tend to be less adventurous in the food department you gotta do whatever works! This is delicious and savory.

Ingredients:

1½ pounds stemmed Concord grapes—antioxidants

1 tablespoon grated orange peel

1 cup water

2½ cups Truvia Baking Blend

½ teaspoon ground cinnamon

½ teaspoon ground cloves (substitute cardamom here if you prefer)

Preparation:

1 Wash the grapes; separate the skins from pulp.

2 Cook the pulp until it's soft; sieve to remove the seeds, if necessary.

3 Add the orange peel and water; cook 10 minutes.

4 Add the skins; heat to boiling.

5 Add the Truvia Baking Blend and spices; cook till thick.

6 Pour hot into sterilized jars. Seal immediately. Let it sit for 24 hours before using.

 Stimulating Cinnamon Facial

Prepare a paste of two parts cinnamon powder and one part honey; leave it on your skin for as long as you can. Rinse off with warm water. Awakens and revitalizes skin.

CUMIN ROASTED CAULIFLOWER
with YOGURT, MINT, and
POMEGRANATE

Makes 4 to 6 Servings

*T*his meal has a Middle Eastern flare; the combo of cumin and pomegranates—spices and seeds—pairs up for a delightfully light but filling dish you could even present as a main course. I find that roasted cauliflower (or any roasted veg) is supremely appetizing, and I could eat it by the bowlful. Cumin and cauliflower are pretty much perfect together.

Ingredients:

2 tablespoons olive oil, divided

1 large head cauliflower, 1 to 1¾ pounds

1 teaspoon whole cumin seeds—digestive and antiseptic

½ teaspoon kosher salt, plus additional

½ teaspoon freshly ground black pepper

1 cup plain yogurt—I use whole-milk yogurt, Greek style

¼ cup crumbled feta (optional)—protein

1 tablespoon chopped fresh mint leaves

½ cup pomegranate seeds—low-cal superfruit

Preparation:

1 Preheat the oven to 425°F. Brush a large baking sheet or roasting pan with 1 tablespoon of the olive oil.

2 Cut your cauliflower into bite-size florets. Toss the florets with the remaining olive oil, cumin seeds, salt, and pepper and spread out on a prepared tray. Roast for 20 to 30 minutes, until the cauliflower is tender and its edges are toasty.

3 Either whisk a pinch of salt into your yogurt, or to make feta-yogurt sauce, blend ¾ cup of yogurt with feta in a food processor until smooth. Spoon yogurt or feta-yogurt sauce onto the cauliflower, then sprinkle the dish with chopped mint and pomegranate seeds.

PASTA with PUMPKIN
MEAT SAUCE

Makes 4 Servings

E very time I make this for dinner my nieces and nephews devour it! The surprise ingredient is pumpkin, which provides a boost of beta-carotene for glowing skin and enhanced immunity. And the best part is, picky-eater kids won't even notice the pumpkin is there. And I sure do know a lot of picky eaters.

Ingredients:

1 package whole wheat rotini pasta or whole wheat penne

1 pound turkey, ground, at least 90 percent lean—lean protein

26 ounces marinara sauce—look for low sodium—vitamins and minerals

½ cup pumpkin purée

1 cup shredded cheese, reduced-fat sharp cheddar or 4-cheese
    Mexican blend

Preparation:

1 Prepare whole wheat rotini or penne pasta according to the box directions, drain, and set aside in a covered pot.

2 Brown the ground turkey meat. When the turkey is cooked through, add the marinara sauce and canned pumpkin purée. Mix thoroughly until bubbly hot.

3 Add the turkey mixture to the pasta and toss. Top with reduced-fat shredded cheddar cheese or 4-cheese Mexican blend. Thoroughly mix until the cheese is melted and blended throughout the pasta.

ASPARAGUS and CHICKEN ENCHILADAS

Makes 12 Enchiladas

*E*nchiladas is Spanish for comfort food. Or, maybe it's Borbafood. Either way, this recipe for tortillas wrapped around a delicious filling is another favorite of mine that I prepare at home often. Asparagus is packed with anti-oxidants, high in fiber, and loaded with age- and disease-fighting vitamins and minerals. This is my go-to dish when I need extra fiber in my diet. The recipe calls for fiber powder, too, which can be "sneaked" into so many recipes to get its benefits. Fiber powder helps draw toxins from the body, thus clarifying and controlling oil on the skin.

Ingredients:

½ cup butter

½ cup all-purpose flour

3 cups chicken broth

8 ounces sour cream—lactic acid

½ cup green taco sauce

1 cup black beans—fiber

12 (8-inch) flour tortillas

12 ounces Monterey Jack cheese, shredded

3 cups cooked and shredded chicken—protein

½ cup finely chopped sweet onion

2½ pounds asparagus, trimmed and blanched—don't precook asparagus for too long; it should still be firm and crisp

2 tablespoons Metamucil fiber powder, unflavored, or the brand of your choice

½ cup grated Parmesan cheese

Tabasco sauce, to taste

1 pink grapefruit, cut in triangular wedges, as garnish

Preparation:

1 Preheat the oven to 425°F. Spray two 9 x 9 glass dishes (or one large 9 x 13 glass dish) with nonstick spray.

2 In a medium saucepan, melt the butter over medium heat. Whisk in the flour and cook, stirring for 1 minute. Gradually add the broth and cook, whisking, until thick (5 minutes). Remove from the heat. Whisk in the sour cream and taco sauce, add the beans, and set aside.

3 Lay out the tortillas on your counter or work surface. Place 2 tablespoons of Jack cheese, ¼ cup of chicken, onions, and asparagus down the center of the tortilla. Spoon 3 tablespoons of sauce on top of the mixture, and sprinkle on the fiber powder. Roll and place seam-down. Place six enchiladas in each dish. Sprinkle with Jack cheese, spoon on extra sauce, top with Parmesan and Tabasco, to taste.

4 Bake for 25 minutes, or until a light golden color and bubbly. Remove from the oven, plate, and serve with a grapefruit wedge.

Fab Fiber

You've probably seen the commercials where the lab-coated doctor recommends "adding more fiber to your diet," but why? If you want great looking healthy skin then getting the right amount of fiber in your diet is essential. Fiber (also known as roughage) eliminates toxins, helps control blood-sugar levels, and can help block bad fats from being absorbed into the bloodstream, just to name a few of its life-essential benefits. High-fiber foods include: fruits such as apples (with the skin), bananas, pears (with the skin), prunes, raspberries, and strawberries; vegetables and greens such as artichokes, broccoli, cauliflower, sweet corn, and turnip greens; grains such as oat bran, oatmeal, pearl barley, and whole wheat products; and seeds and nuts such as almonds, pistachios (and their skins), and sunflower seeds.

SHRIMP BBQ

Makes 5 Servings

This is a simple recipe that yields head-to-toe skin benefits, especially from the high protein content, vitamin C, and antioxidants. The vitamin E is a natural preservative that also acts as an anti-inflammatory emollient and protects against free radical damage. This dish is especially great for aging skin.

Ingredients:

20 large shrimp—protein

1 cup olive oil

Juice of 3 lemons

¼ cup low-sodium soy sauce

¼ cup finely chopped parsley

¼ cup lychee syrup with pulp solids

3 tablespoons chopped fresh tarragon—essential oils

Preparation:

1 Use cooking scissors to cut down the back of each shrimp shell and remove the black vein, keeping the shell intact. (Alternately, when you buy shrimp from the fishmonger, you can request that they be "cleaned.") Wash the shrimp thoroughly and place in a large bowl.

2 Pour the olive oil, lemon juice, soy sauce, parsley, lychee syrup, and tarragon over the shrimp. Let the shrimp stand for 2 hours, tossing occasionally to marinate equally. Refrigerate.

3 Heat up the grill while the shrimp are marinating.

4 Arrange the shrimp in basket grills, or thread through skewers, and cook over hot barbecue coals for 5 to 6 minutes, turning twice. The shrimp should be tender and moist with charred shells.

CRANBERRY SHRIMP COCKTAIL

Makes 12 Servings

Every day, our skin is under assault—from UV rays, pollution, or cigarette smoke, for example. That damage causes free radicals, which are oxygen molecules that have lost an electron. The result is visible skin damage, in the form of lines, wrinkles, and redness. Luckily, antioxidants can supply those missing electrons, calm attacking molecules, and prevent damage. And cranberries provide us with antioxidants. In fact, antioxidants are among the most important preventive ingredients in the skin-care arsenal.

Ingredients: Cocktail sauce

1 (14-ounce) can jellied cranberry sauce—antioxidant benefits
½ cup chile sauce
2 tablespoons finely chopped onion
2 tablespoons Worcestershire sauce
2 tablespoons red wine vinegar
1 teaspoon prepared horseradish—potent gastric stimulant; aids in digestion
1 pink grapefruit, peeled, and sectioned with skin and white fibers removed
Pink grapefruit slices, as garnish

Shrimp

48 cooked, medium, shelled, and deveined shrimp with tails left on
   (about 1 pound)

Preparation: Cocktail sauce

1 Combine all sauce ingredients in a medium saucepan. Bring to a boil on medium-high heat.

2 Reduce the heat; simmer for 10 minutes or until the onion is tender and the sauce thickens slightly, stirring frequently.

3 Cool; refrigerate until cold.

4 Fill a large bowl with crushed ice; place the bowl of cocktail sauce in the center of the ice.

Shrimp

Arrange the shrimp and pink grapefruit slices on crushed ice around the bowl of sauce.

YEAR-ROUND
MINESTRONE SOUP

A savory, steaming hot soup is replenishing, satisfying, and good for the soul. This one happens to be great for skin clarity, too, due to its superfoods and decidedly healthy ingredients. Cannellini beans are very popular in Italian cuisine; their low cost, long shelf life, and gastronomic versatility make them useful in any kitchen. This recipe uses the canned variety. If you already have them raw in your pantry and prefer to use those, take note that when soaked, they double in size—so less beans go a long way. Here's a hearty meal that's low in calories and high in taste. You may even want to double the ingredients to make enough soup to freeze and save for a rainy day.

Ingredients:

2 tablespoons extra-virgin olive oil—skin soother

1 medium zucchini, diced—high in manganese, good for wound healing

1 medium sweet potato, diced—superfood

1 large carrot, diced

1 small onion, finely diced

2 cloves garlic, minced

32-ounce carton vegetable broth

16 ounces tomato sauce—lycopene

1 box seashell pasta

1 teaspoon ground cumin—antibacterial properties for skin

1 (16-ounce) can cannellini beans, drained and rinsed

3 sprigs fresh thyme

1 tablespoon honey—skin saver

Salt and freshly ground black pepper, to taste

4 shakes Tabasco sauce, or hot sauce of choice

Parmesan cheese, to taste

¼ cup cut, loosely packed fresh basil (optional)

Preparation:

1 Heat the oil in a large saucepan over medium-high heat.

2 Add the zucchini, sweet potato, carrot, onion, garlic, and cook. Stir frequently until the vegetables start to soften, about 10 minutes. (You may want to use a spatter guard against the oil.)

3 Stir in the broth, tomato sauce, pasta shells, and cumin; cover, and bring to a boil.

4 Add the beans and thyme. Cook, uncovered, at a low boil until the pasta is done, about 10 minutes.

5 Remove the thyme sprigs, add the honey, and season with salt and pepper, to taste.

6 Serve in individual bowls and top with Tabasco, Parmesan cheese, and basil (optional).

 TIP: For treating the T-zone, muddle (mash/mix together) the basil in a small bowl and then place on the T-zone for about 1 minute. Rinse off. This should keep the oil zone balanced all day.

Spud Power

Sweet potatoes are a superfood that should be enjoyed with meals year-round. Sweet potatoes are packed with beta-carotene, an antioxidant that fights aging. Beta-carotene also balances your skin's pH, helps combat dryness, and promotes cell turnover—all resulting in smoother skin. Try these tubers cut up and roasted with herbs or onions for an easy, savory side dish. Or roasted and doused in cinnamon plus a sprinkle of brown sugar, if you want to go the sweet route. I love sweet and savory everything.

TURKEY BURGER SLIDERS
and YOGURT SAUCE

Makes 8 Mini-Sliders

This recipe uses cumin, a distinct spice present in almost every Indian dish. Cumin is rich in vitamin E, a nutrient widely known for its ability to rejuvenate skin. Middle Eastern and Mexican cuisines use a lot of cumin, too, perhaps because of its pungent flavor, or for its amazing antiseptic properties. Cumin is high in iron and is good for the digestive system. Many people mix cumin with warm water and drink it at night as a tea to curb digestive troubles. Cumin is high in antioxidants, such as vitamin C and vitamin A, which provide numerous benefits to the skin. The antiseptic properties help fight infection and make cumin a useful treatment for skin challenges. In this recipe, its nutty, peppery flavor adds zing to the turkey meat. Turkey meat is a good blank canvas for spicing and tastes delicious with a spike of cumin. Selenium is another superfood your skin needs to thrive. Whole wheat breads, turkey, and Brazil nuts are great sources of selenium.

Ingredients: Burger

1 pound ground turkey—protein

½ teaspoon rock salt

¼ teaspoon ground black pepper

1 tablespoon crushed Brazil nuts

Tabasco, to taste—capsaicin

Pinch cumin powder

1 teaspoon extra-virgin olive oil

Sauce

1½ cups plain nonfat Greek yogurt—a favorite among athletes and healthy eaters

¼ cup shredded cucumber—hydration

2 teaspoons chopped fresh dill

1½ teaspoons Dijon mustard—high in selenium

1 teaspoon garlic powder

4 whole wheat rolls, split

2 avocados, cut into wedges, as garnish

Preparation:

1 In a medium-size bowl, gently mix the turkey, salt, pepper, crushed nuts, Tabasco, and cumin.

2 Form the mixture into eight balls. Flatten into patties, about 1-inch thick.

3 In a large skillet over medium-high heat, warm the oil.

4 Add the burgers and cook for 5 to 6 minutes per side, figure 5 minutes for every 1 inch of thickness.

5 While the burgers cook, mix the yogurt, cucumber, dill, mustard, and garlic powder in a small bowl.

6 Dollop the sauce on top of each burger, cap with a bun, and serve with a wedge of avocado.

♪ Home-Spa Greek Yogurt Facial with Mustard and Cumin

Freeze the yogurt until firm and very cold. Fold in the mustard and cumin with the yogurt. Apply to face. The cold helps with facial puffiness; yogurt hyperhydrates and balances texture and tone. Cumin acts as an antimicrobial agent to clarify skin. Mustard helps stimulate circulation and gently exfoliates dead skin cells. Exfoliation plays an important role in skin's youthful appearance, as it rids the skin of dull, dead skin cells. Cell turnover in young, supple skin takes anywhere from 7 to 14 days; turnover in mature skin can take up to a month.

♪ Yogurt-Honey-Lemon Facial for Sensitive Skin

If you don't feel like cooking tonight but want to treat your face right, try this sensitive-skin facial. Plain acidophilus yogurt helps restore a supportive bacterial environment for sensitive or enflamed skin, and mixing it with honey and lemon moisturizes and leaves skin smooth with shrunken pores. Apply a thin layer of this natural concoction to your face. Let it dry and leave on for up to 1 hour. So easy to look beautiful!

AVOCADO-GRAPEFRUIT RELISH

*T*his is a basic recipe I literally thought of while gazing into my refrigerator's crisper drawer. It's easy to get creative when you let yourself flow!

Ingredients:

1 large ripe avocado

½ pink grapefruit

1 clove garlic

½ bunch cilantro

Preparation:

Place all the ingredients in a food processor, pulse for 5 seconds. Serve cold.

 Avocado Smoothing Facial

An avocado mask can improve very dry skin, smoothing your skin to its natural supple state. Smash 1/2 of an avocado until whipped, and apply a thin layer to your face, avoiding the eye area. Rinse with warm water and then a splash of cold water to close the pores.

APPLE and KIELBASA SALAD

Makes 1 Serving

*T*his is a wonderful cooked salad with multiple skin-care benefits. There's nothing like warm fruit, and the meeting of sweet with salty is one of my favorite combos. Kielbasa is Polish for "sausage," and it's usually preflavored with garlic, pimento, and cloves, but your butcher may sell something different. You can purchase it in thick 2-inch diameter links. Oftentimes it's also sold precooked and only needs to be heated before serving. Be sure to find out if yours is precooked as this will effect cooking time.

Ingredients:

4 tablespoons cider vinegar—good for acne

1 tablespoon grainy mustard—combo of honey, turmeric, garlic, and brown sugar so good for you

1 teaspoon Truvia Baking Blend

⅛ teaspoon kosher salt

¼ teaspoon black pepper

3 tablespoons extra-virgin olive oil

¾ pound turkey kielbasa, sliced

1 (10-ounce package) shredded red cabbage—helps lower cholesterol

3 Granny Smith apples, cored and grated—fiber

½ teaspoon caraway seeds—essential oils, antioxidants, fiber

1 pink grapefruit, cut into triangles

Preparation:

1 In a small bowl, mix together 2 tablespoons of the cider vinegar, the mustard, Truvia Baking Blend, salt, and pepper.

2 Whisk in the oil until blended. Set the dressing aside.

3 Coat a large skillet with cooking spray. Heat over medium-high heat. Add the sliced kielbasa. Cook for 4 minutes, turning until browned. If you purchased precooked kielbasa, cut the cooking time in the skillet by half.

4 Remove to a plate. Add the cabbage, apples, remaining 2 tablespoons of cider vinegar, and caraway seeds to the skillet. Cook for 4 minutes. Remove from the heat, stir in the kielbasa and dressing. Toss gently to coat. Serve with the grapefruit triangles.

MOUTHWATERING GRAPEFRUIT MERINGUE

Makes 4 Servings

I find grapefruit to be a real thirst quencher. Something about the acidity and lightly sour taste makes it one of the most invigorating citrus fruits that's pure and revitalizing. To up the deliciousness even more, I've morphed it into a refreshing meringue that caps a warmed grapefruit. Making a great meringue seems to be one of the mysteries of life: Everyone has a different theory on how to do it, when to add what ingredients, and what kinds of external effects—humidity, for example—can kink up the process. Below is my recommendation, but tweak it as you see fit if you know your meringue method to be tried and true.

Ingredients:

3 egg whites, room temperature—a lower-cholesterol protein
¼ teaspoon cream of tartar—can help with nicotine withdrawal
1 teaspoon vanilla extract
¼ teaspoon salt
¼ cup confectionary Truvia Baking Blend
2 large pink grapefruits, halved, sections precut for easier eating—
    potassium source

Preparation:

1 Preheat the oven to 350°F. Place the egg whites in a small bowl and add a pinch of tartar. Let the tartar settle in; this will help to strengthen the egg whites for forming peaks later.

2 Next, use an electric mixer to beat the egg whites with the vanilla, cream of tartar, and salt until foamy. (Take care to assure that all utensils and the bowl are very clean. Any greasy residue can inhibit texture.)

3 Gradually add the confectionary Truvia Baking Blend and continue beating until the mixture is shiny and forms stiff peaks. Cover the entire open-face surface of each grapefruit half with generous gobs of meringue.

4 Bake for 15 or 20 minutes until lightly browned. Serve immediately.

PRUNE, CRANBERRY, and WALNUT STUFFING

Makes 12 (½-Cup) Servings

E ven though we sometimes associate them with Grannie's delight, prunes are simply dried plums sans pit. They are highly antioxidant (and yes, they are a natural laxative) and offer protection against osteoporosis. They are high in soluble fiber and vitamin K, which works toward bone strength. Their deep sweet taste and sticky texture make them wonderful to cook with for sweet or savory dishes.

Ingredients:

½ cup butter or margarine

1 cup dried cranberries—can help strengthen the immune system

1 cup chopped prunes

1 cup chopped apples, with skin on or peeled—fiber

1 cup chopped walnuts—antioxidant rich

1½ cups apple juice

1 cup chopped parsley

1 box (two 6-ounce bags) seasoned breadcrumb mix

Preparation:

1 Preheat the oven to 350°F.

2 Combine the butter or margarine, fruits, and nuts, and stir the apple juice in gradually. Add the parsley and breadcrumb mix.

3 Spoon into a 2½- or 3-quart greased casserole dish. Bake, covered, for 30 minutes.

4 Remove the cover and bake for 5 to 10 minutes longer for a crisper top.

PEANUT TOFU WRAP

*A*n *easy-to-assemble healthy, crunchy power snack with protein, vitamins A and C, and iron. I try to be mindful when eating peanuts as allergies to them are so prevalent nowadays and we never know if the person sitting next to us could have a bad reaction, even from the scent of the nuts.*

Ingredients:

2 tablespoons store-bought Thai peanut sauce

2 (8-inch) whole wheat flour tortillas

4 ounces thinly sliced seasoned baked tofu—soy

½ cup sliced red bell pepper—antioxidant

16 thinly sliced snow peas

Preparation:

Spread peanut sauce on each tortilla. Place tofu, peppers, and snow peas in the center; fold the sides over the filling and roll up. There you have it!

One-Two Punch: Polyphenols and Flavonoids!

Antioxidants are a daily necessity internally and externally. For the one-two punch against aging, you should have a combination of polyphenols (a more potent antioxidant found in Acai and dark berries) along with high levels of flavonoids (found in nutrient-rich darker fruits and vegetables). When you combine these ingredients topically and internally, all the layers of skin have the potential to communicate, promoting healthier looking, ageless skin.

CREAMLESS CREAM of ASPARAGUS SOUP

Makes 8 Servings

This recipe is gluten-, dairy-, and soy-free. But it's rich in vitamins and minerals that are hydrating and good for your complexion. This soup gets its creaminess from coconut—a natural, delicious alternative to wheat and grain that's packed with dietary fiber and is a good source of protein. I love anything that tastes like cream; I should have been French. The best way to derive the health-giving gifts of coconut is to use virgin coconut oil. It's a small investment in your health that yields tremendous returns.

Ingredients:

½ medium white onion, chopped—chromium; needed to help regulate blood sugar
2 cloves garlic, crushed
1 teaspoon virgin coconut oil—rich in polyphenols
1 (24-ounce) carton low-sodium chicken stock
1½ pounds asparagus
5 to 6 new potatoes—complex carbohydrates
Salt and pepper, to taste
2 teaspoons raw coconut flour—gluten-free

Preparation:

1 Sauté the onions and garlic in a stockpot on medium heat with the coconut oil. Add the carton of chicken stock.

2 Snap off the tough ends of the asparagus, then chop into 1-inch sections and add to the chicken stock.

3 Cut the new potatoes into quarters and add to the pot. Season with salt and pepper, to taste. Bring to a boil, then turn to low and set on simmer for 1 to 2 hours until the asparagus is very soft.

4 Remove the potatoes from the pot and set aside. Use a blender to cream the broth and asparagus mixture—let the broth cool a bit before blending. When the asparagus and broth are blended thoroughly, add the potatoes back into the pot and turn up the heat to almost boiling.

5 Add 2 teaspoons of raw coconut flour to the pot and whisk until it's combined. Add as much coconut flour as you like until the soup is as thick as you want it.

GRILLED ASPARAGUS SPEARS with SMOKED SALMON and TANGY MUSTARD

*E*ating asparagus is a health-smart move. More calories will be burned to digest it than gained from eating it and its skin-care benefits are many. Smoked salmon is more than a bagel topping or an omelet filling. It doesn't lose its health benefits in the smoking process and is super easy to prepare and cook with because it is already cooked! It is low in fat and high in protein, and a good source of phosphorous, selenium, and zinc. I always have thin slices of it in my refrigerator, which I pick up from my local deli on the weekend. When I don't have the time to prepare a proper meal, I finesse a piece of smoked salmon into a hand roll, and snack on it when I need energy. Sometimes I just wrap it around a cheese stick, munch, and go.

Ingredients:

1½ pounds asparagus, tough ends cut off

4 teaspoons extra-virgin olive oil

Truffle sea salt (can purchase online) and freshly ground pepper, to taste

6 thin slices smoked salmon (about 4 ounces), each cut in 4 lengthwise strips—protein; vitamin E

2 tablespoons Tangy Mustard Dressing (see recipe on page 103)

Cilantro sprigs, as garnish—a natural cleansing agent

Preparation:

1 Preheat the grill to medium-high heat.

2 Lightly coat the asparagus with the oil. Season with salt and pepper, to taste.

3 Grill fo,r 3 minutes, or until al dente but not soft. Remove from the grill. The asparagus will continue to cook as they cool. Do not overcook the spears.

4 When cool enough to handle, wrap each spear with a slice of the salmon. Arrange on a serving platter and drizzle with the Tangy Mustard Dressing. Garnish with cilantro and serve immediately, or chill to serve later.

TANGY MUSTARD DRESSING

Makes 1½ Cups

Mustard is a good-for-you condiment. And here's why: It contains phytonutrients—natural chemicals derived from plant foods, which can help prevent disease and keep the body working well. Mustard is also rich in selenium and magnesium, two "miracle minerals" that have anti-inflammatory properties. Mustard seeds come from the mustard plant, which is a cruciferous veggie related to broccoli, Brussels sprouts, and cabbage. Of course you'd have to eat massive quantities of mustard to get the maximum benefits, but eating it daily—in sauces, as a condiment, and so forth—is a great start. Green veggies and other root vegetables, like radishes, are fat-burning foods that help kick-start the body into losing weight. These appetite suppressants are free-radical "scavengers" that help flush toxins from your body.

Ingredients:

½ cup silken tofu—low cal, high calcium

¼ cup white miso (purchase at an Asian foods market, or in gourmet foods area of supermarket)

¼ cup unseasoned rice wine vinegar

¼ cup spicy mustard

¼ cup fresh lemon juice

1 tablespoon Truvia Baking Blend

2 cloves garlic

½ teaspoon Sriracha (purchase at an Asian foods market, or in gourmet foods area of supermarket)

½ teaspoon Worcestershire sauce

¼ teaspoon ground black pepper

Preparation:

Combine all the ingredients in a blender or food processor until smooth.

LENTIL SLOPPY JOES

Makes 4 Servings

Hero Recipe!

Another excellent source of fiber in an American classic sandwich. Joes always remind me of school cafeterias and summer camp. There was always something wonderfully fun about getting to eat a burger/sandwich that was messy by design. This version uses lentils in place of ground beef so you can up your health intake while lowering your calorie count. Lentil-buying tip: Whether you purchase lentils prepackaged or in bulk, look for those that appear largely unbroken (bags with broken lentils appear "dusty"). Buy from a source that has a good turnover. Sort through lentils before cooking them to remove any small stones or twigs. Spreading them out on a platter of a contrasting color will make this task easier.

Ingredients:

1 cup lentils, green
1 tablespoon olive oil
1 medium yellow onion, diced
1 medium green bell pepper, diced—nutrient-dense
2 cloves garlic, minced
3 tablespoons chile powder
2 teaspoons dried oregano—good for acne treatment program; high in vitamin K
½ teaspoon kosher salt
1 (8-ounce) can tomato sauce, preferably no-salt-added
¼ cup tomato paste
3 tablespoons maple syrup
1 tablespoon yellow mustard—anti-inflammatory properties
4 whole wheat rolls, toasted (optional, for serving)

Preparation:

1 Combine the lentils and 4 cups of water in a large saucepan. Cover the pan and bring the water to a boil. Reduce the heat to low and simmer for about 25 minutes, until the lentils are tender. Drain and set aside.

2 Heat the olive oil in a medium pot over medium-high heat. Add the onion and bell pepper and sauté until softened, about 7 minutes. Add the garlic and sauté for 1 minute. Add the cooked lentils, chile powder, oregano, and salt. Add the tomato sauce and tomato paste and mix well. Reduce the heat to low and simmer for 10 minutes.

3 Add the maple syrup and mustard and heat through. Turn off the heat and let the lentil mixture sit for about 10 minutes, allowing the flavors to meld. Spoon the mixture over toasted buns, if desired.

Tomato Paste Acne Cream

Tomatoes have more nutritional value once cooked—the antioxidant becomes more bioavailable to our bodies when heated or cooked, so our bodies can absorb it more. Thus, using a tomato paste has more benefits than using a raw tomato. Mix together ¼ cup of low-sodium tomato paste, 1 teaspoon of olive oil, and enough apple cider vinegar to make a smooth paste. Apply as a mask on neck and face to alleviate acne. Leave on for 15 minutes and then gently rinse off with warm water. Finally, splash some cold water on your face to close your pores.

Drink some of that apple cider vinegar, too! It has a natural effect of removing toxins from your body.

FRESH ZUCCHINI PANCAKES

Makes 6 Pancakes

The first time I ate these savory 'cakes I was on a ski trip in Utah. My group was at a snowy roadside diner and these were on the breakfast special menu. We needed to tank up on solid energy food for a full day on the slopes, and zucchini is high in vitamin C, which helps water flow to the skin. I have since made them pretty much whenever I make pancakes for brunch. At home, I use whole wheat for my pancake batter, which is not called for in this recipe, but you certainly can use it instead of the biscuit mix.

Ingredients:

⅔ cup biscuit mix

5 rounded teaspoons Metamucil fiber powder

¼ teaspoon pepper

¼ cup grated Parmesan cheese

1 medium zucchini, thinly grated—cholesterol-lowering superfood

1 cup grated cheddar cheese

2 eggs—protein

½ cup buttermilk—the higher acid in buttermilk makes it taste better in
   these pancakes

Spray butter, to taste

1 cup sour cream, as topping—lactic acid, great for smooth skin

Preparation:

Mix together all the ingredients in the order listed with a wooden spoon. Save the spray butter for the griddle and flavoring at the end. Spoon the mixture in pancake-size dollops onto the spray-buttered hot griddle. Brown one side and then turn and brown the other side. Serve hot with a dollop of sour cream.

MOM'S ZUCCHINI BREAD

Makes 2 Loaves

I love sweets that have a smart side. I'm all about comfort food with a beauty benefit and this bread served warm with a pat of butter (or not!) is simply heavenly. Truffle butter and jalapeño butter are awesome, too, and I recommend you buy them for your refrigerator condiment section.

Ingredients:

3 cups all-purpose flour

1 teaspoon salt

1 teaspoon baking powder

1 teaspoon baking soda

3 teaspoons ground cinnamon

3 eggs

1 cup vegetable oil

2¼ cups Truvia Baking Blend

3 teaspoons vanilla extract

2 cups grated zucchini—incredibly low in calories plus major hydration

1 cup chopped walnuts

Preparation:

1 Grease and flour two 8 x 4-inch pans. Preheat the oven to 325°F.

2 Sift the flour, salt, baking powder, baking soda, and cinnamon together in a bowl.

3 Beat the eggs, oil, Truvia Baking Blend, and vanilla together in a large bowl. Add the sifted ingredients to the creamed mixture, and beat well. Stir in the zucchini and nuts until well combined. Pour the batter into the prepared pans.

4 Bake for 40 to 60 minutes, or until a tester inserted in the center comes out clean.

5 Cool in the pan on a rack for 20 minutes. Remove the bread from the pan and completely cool.

GRILLED BEEF BRACCIOLE

Makes 2 Servings

M y nieces call this delicious dish "roll-up steak," and, for children, I have learned, anything with a theme or a twist gets them eating the healthy stuff. Start off here by preheating the grill.

Ingredients:

2 pounds round steak, flattened to ¼-inch thickness

¼ cup olive oil

Salt and pepper, enough for seasoning and to taste

¼ cup grated pecorino Romano or feta

¼ cup finely chopped parsley—anti-inflammatory properties; boosts
  immune system

2 tablespoons finely chopped, fresh oregano leaves

4 cloves garlic, crushed—cancer fighter!

Butcher's twine

Preparation:

1 Brush the steak on the faceup side with 2 tablespoons of oil, then season with salt and pepper.

2 Combine the cheese, parsley, oregano, and garlic in a small bowl. Sprinkle the cheese mixture evenly over the steak.

3 Starting with the long end, roll the meat up and tie it with butcher's twine.

4 Brush the entire roll with oil, and season with salt and pepper.

5 Place the meat on the grill, seam-side up, and grill for about 10 to 12 minutes, rotating until golden brown on all sides.

6 Remove and let rest for 10 minutes before slicing.

RED PALM OIL FISH STEW
with VEGGIES

Makes 2 Servings

Hero Recipe!

This meal uses the latest beauty discovery—red palm oil. Red palm oil has been used traditionally in African-inspired dishes for centuries, but only as of recently are we starting to learn more about it and see its health benefits. Rich in vitamins A and E, I like to think of red palm oil as "the new Argan oil." Red palm oil comes from the same part of the palm tree as regular palm oil, but it's less processed and retains the red color from its high concentration of carotenes. Try to incorporate red palm oil in many of your dishes . . . start with a few shakes and build from there. This recipe comes from Juka's Palm Oil brand, inspired by my friend Juka Ceesay.

Ingredients:

2 pounds fish (filet or whole fish of choice)
1 Maggi Seasoning Cube
Pinch of salt, to taste
½ teaspoon black pepper
2 tablespoons chopped garlic
¾ cup red palm oil (find in the ethnic foods aisle, or online)
3 medium-size onions, chopped
3 medium-size tomatoes
2 tablespoons tomato paste
1 bunch scallions
1 teaspoon of soy sauce (optional)
½ habañero pepper (optional)
¾ cup water
½ lemon

Preparation:

1 Remove the skin from the fish and rinse to clean.

2 Season the cleaned fish with ½ of the Maggi Seasoning Cube, salt, black pepper, and ½ tablespoon of garlic.

3 Heat the oil for 2 minutes and then sauté the fish until browned on both sides. (You can also bake the fish in the oven.) Remove the fish, reserving the oil.

4 Using the reserved oil, sauté the onions, tomatoes, tomato paste, remaining garlic, scallions, the remaining ½ of the Maggi Seasoning Cube, soy sauce, and the habañero pepper (optional) for 20 minutes, until the liquid has completely evaporated. (Let it reduce down until it turns into somewhat of a paste: this is the secret of the dish.)

5 Add the fish back to the pan and add the water, lemon, and salt, to taste. Cook on medium heat until the fish is cooked through (generally 10 to 15 minutes).

TIP: A natural antibiotic, garlic is one of nature's strongest medicines. Whether you bake it, sauté it, eat it raw, or put it in your socks, it will help your immune system year-round. At the first signs of a cold or fever, I thinly slice four garlic cloves and place two in each sock and go to sleep with socks on. The body absorbs the garlic through the pores and helps generate sweat—good for getting rid of colds and toxins.

FISH and KALE with RED PALM OIL

Makes 2 Servings

Hero Recipe!

This simple recipe is bursting with ingredients that boost beauty. It is also from Juka's Palm Oil brand, inspired by my friend Juka Ceesay.

Ingredients:

1½ pounds fish fillet

1 pinch salt

1 teaspoon lemon juice

½ cup red palm oil

1 large white onion, chopped

1 bundle scallions, chopped

1 teaspoon chopped garlic

½ habañero pepper, to taste, optional

1 teaspoon chopped ginger

1 handful cherry tomatoes

1 Maggi Seasoning Cube

2 handfuls mushrooms

2 handfuls kale

Preparation:

1 Clean the fish and season with the salt and lemon juice.

2 Add the palm oil into a heated pot for 2 seconds and add the seasoned fish right away. Sauté the fish on both sides for 4 minutes at a time or until semidone. Then remove the fish from the pot.

3 Add the chopped onions, chopped scallions, garlic, habañero pepper, chopped ginger, cherry tomatoes, Maggi Cube, and a pinch of salt to taste. Mix the ingredients and let them sauté for 5 minutes.

4 Add the sautéed fish back in the pot on top of everything; put the mushrooms and kale on top of the fish and mix in slightly. Cover and cook for 4 minutes.

Kale Scrub

Mince 5 cleaned kale leaves in a food processor, or by hand. Mix some vegetable shortening into the minced kale and apply from neck to toes prior to showering. (The vegetable shortening is the binder to make the kale stick to your skin. Otherwise, you are just rubbing minced greens on your skin and hoping for the best.) Allow up to 15 minutes for the scrub to set, then lather and rinse off with warm water. If you do not use vegetable shortening in your home, you can combine the minced kale with any moisturizing lotion.

Home-Spa Pimple-Crushing Facial

Mix 1 tablespoon of apple cider vinegar or white vinegar into 1 cup of warm water. Stir. Dip a cotton ball into the mix and gently dab on the face. This is an easy, antibacterial at-home treatment.

Fruit-Enzyme Facial for Fighting Brown Spots

Mash strawberries, peeled fresh apricots, and lemon juice together to make a paste. Apply to your face to get rid of brown spots and freckling. Leave it on for 15 minutes and then rinse off with tepid water.

Facial Mist for Rosy Cheeks

Green tea is an anti-inflammatory with healing properties. Rosewater is derived from the natural beauty and healing power of the rose. Rosewater aids with circulation and has value as a toning astringent. To make this facial mist, steep a green tea bag in hot water and allow it to cool. Using a plastic bottle mister, add tea and rose water in a 1:1 ratio. Use as an astringent mist on a clean face before applying moisturizer.

Jojoba and Essential Oils Facial for Lackluster Skin

To restore vibrancy to lackluster skin, mix jojoba oil with essential oils of evening primrose, lavender, rosemary, and thyme. Essential oils help soften and reconstruct cellular bonds; jojoba helps restore skin's protective hydrolipidic film. Apply thin layer for 10 minutes; remove with tissue or warm cloth.

I Get Misty

Misting your skin often is, in my opinion, the critical capture of hydrated, glowing skin. Take this one seriously because it couldn't be more true: You only have one face. You can love it and lavish goodness upon it, or leave it be. My recommendation is to be diligent day, night, and when tired to make certain you spray-mist your skin if you're not washing and moisturizing before you go to bed. The results are so worth it.

Got Bac-ne?

If you frequent nightclubs and restaurants—and who says you shouldn't?—know that the booths you sit in harbor tons of bacteria. If you are wearing a sleeveless dress, open-back blouse, short-sleeve shirt, or any other garment where your skin is making contact with the booth, you are susceptible to picking up germs and bacteria that could potentially clog pores and irritate your skin—hence, back acne. Ever notice how the booth sometimes feels sticky? Think about it: Most establishments are not wiping down these oft-used seating areas nearly as often as you would at home. Take care to do so with an antibacterial wipe, or put a couple of squirts of antibacterial lotion on a napkin (cloth is best) and quickly wipe down where you will sit. I always carry a small bottle of antibacterial lotion in my bag. Much more useful than the pens floating around in there that I never seem to write with nowadays! Also, if you're out on the town or clubbing and need to remove excess shine, a new sanitary toilet sheet cover will absorb oil like a sponge.

TIP: Reducing irritation is important in clearing back acne. But let's face it, you must sit in chairs and wear clothes, so something will be touching your back pretty much all the time. Backpacks, in particular, can create more direct and ongoing irritation, which may aggravate back acne in some people. They also stifle airflow, which is needed to heal wounds. Try carrying your gear in something other than a backpack.

Fruits + Veggies = The Skinny

Very low-calorie or negative-calorie foods include apples, broccoli, carrots, cauliflower, celery, endive, grapefruit, hot chile peppers, lemon, lettuce, onion, oranges, strawberries, tangerines, tomatoes, watermelon, zucchini, and cucumbers. Get chomping! Cucumbers are also easy on the eyes . . . excellent for reducing swelling and softening skin tissue around the delicate eye area. Cukes are a rich source of silica, a trace mineral that strengthens skin's connective tissue. You can slice cucumbers thin and rub them all over your skin for a refreshing pick-me-up that's soothing and healing, too.

Worth Its Salt

There are literally hundreds of uses for this magical salt named after a bitter saline spring at Epsom in Surrey, England. Epsom salt can soothe the body, relax the nervous system, cure skin problems, soothe back pain and aching limbs, ease muscle strain, heal cuts, treat colds, exfoliate skin, work with hair treatments, and draw toxins from the body. One of the simplest ways to benefit from it—and draw muscle pain from your body—is to soak in a tubful of hot water with a few cups of Epsom salt added. I did this after a three-mile run and my body felt great the next day—not sore at all. Epsom salt is also antibacterial, making it great for a foot soak, too.

Try these other Epsom salt home-spa treatments:

- **Epsom Exfoliating Face Cleanser.** To clean your face and exfoliate skin at the same time, mix ½ teaspoon of Epsom salt with your regular cleansing cream. Gently massage it into the skin and rinse with cold water. You'll really feel your skin opening up and getting smoother beneath your very fingertips.

- **Epsom Blackhead Remover.** Add 1 teaspoon of Epsom salt and 3 drops of iodine to ½ cup of boiling water. Apply this mixture to the blackheads with a cotton ball.

- **Epsom Facial.** Mix ½ teaspoon of Epsom salt with cleansing cream for deep-pore cleansing. Massage on the skin, rinse with cool water, and pat dry.

Vitamin C Skin-Care Treatment—Inside and Outside

If you want to get a double bang out of your vitamin C buck, you need to eat it *and* put it on your skin. This will offer you maximum absorption. Vitamin C will help kill bacteria on the skin and break up greasy, waxy deposits. Vitamin C enhances collagen production and repair when used topically. Vitamin C is an antioxidant that can decrease fine wrinkles and age spots and increase hydration. Pick up a bottle of liquid vitamin C from your health food store or purchase one online. Amazon.com sells it and so do many other sites. Ester C is what you should be looking for topically and internally. Liquid vitamin C is great to use in cooking, beverages, and topically as a serum. Read package directions and be careful with how much you take as too much can irritate the stomach due to the acidity.

Sound Sleep

Protect your face from the constant cycle of dead skin it sheds and trapped oil, dirt, and bacteria. Change your pillowcases a few times a week. Oils in your hair and residue from hair products rub off on your pillowcases. While you are sleeping, the pores on your face are absorbing everything that's on your pillows. Cotton sheets breathe better for your skin, which helps fight aging, and cotton is a great oil absorber for acnaic skin. If you can invest in high thread-count sheets, they are more absorbent and actually can better protect your skin. Cotton sheets are especially good for teenage skin. If you can see a silhouette on your sheet or pillowcases it's time to change sheets. Your face deserves a fresh environment to lay your tired head.

Luscious Lips Treatment

Freckling, chapped lips, or even sun blisters can occur in the summer heat. In the winter, we experience chapping, flaking, and dryness. To restore moisture to dry lips, purée ⅓ of a peeled cucumber to extract the juice. Pour this into 1 tablespoon of honey and 1 tablespoon of plain yogurt then stir until your balm is blended. Apply like lip gloss and allow it to absorb into your lips. Of course it's edible, but treat your lips, don't eat it!

Into the Core

Chapter 4

In putting this book together, I consulted other experts, industry professionals, friends, and relatives. You can always learn from the people in your life. One of the best zingers of insight I received was from, not surprisingly, my seventy-year-old mother. She said, "Because I am not besieged with major skin problems and lucked out even as a teenager, I have to conclude that having firm and radiant skin must have something to do with my eating patterns. As a young person, I was not privy to unlimited junk food like kids are today. There were no vending machines and the concept of the drive-thru restaurant was quite the novelty. Although I did have my share of ice cream and cheeseburgers, for the most part I grew up in a household that ran its kitchen on fresh ingredients from local markets; my family even knew the people who ran them. We didn't 'order in,' I cooked from scratch and never went a night without my cucumber eye mask and yogurt face pack."

She was gorgeous from the inside out. And still is.

Taking mi madre's experience to heart, I realize that her lifestyle then is less common now. Today's time crush of raising a family, managing a career, and/or running a household offset by readily available feel-good foods can derail any of us at any given time. But unhealthy body fat can *damage organs and muscles,* not just affect the waistline. I think of "core" as not only the center of the body—the hub of physical strength—but as the zone of digestive health. You may be swamped with work, childcare responsibilities, and an overall lack of time to exercise and prepare foods that power your body. This chapter's recipes target core body needs to fuel a healthy digestive system—the core of your bodily functions. I think it's important to note that what we eat and put in and on our bodies should be unilateral considerations.

Additionally, I can't say enough about the power of exercise on the mind, body, and spirit. You simply have to get your body moving, your sweat salting, and your endorphins pumping. Personally, I find the quickest, most effective exercise to be running. If I can crank out a 20-minute run two or three times a week, I can keep my 6-pack from becoming a 2-liter. Please get out there and honor thy body!! If running is not your thing due to feet, knee, or back problems, brisk walking—with hills—is also a great fat burner. You simply have got to sweat. Now onward, my friend!

TOP 5 SVB's Top Five Heroes for Core Health

Whole Wheat—contains all three layers of the grain, increasing vitamins, minerals, and healthy phytochemical intake.

Nuts—heart-healthy Brazil nuts and walnuts are especially good fats your body needs for energy and protein.

Tomatoes—contain vitamins, minerals, and nutrients that balance fluids and contribute to normal digestive functioning.

Green Beans—eaten raw, they increase dietary fiber, fluoride, magnesium, and vitamin A.

Berries (also watermelon)—antioxidant polyphenols create a heart-healthy environment.

HONEY-WHEAT BREAD

Makes 2 Loaves

W*hy not make a tender wheat loaf like the one you might find at a country fair, or cooling on the windowsill at Grandma's? Comfort food that's good for you is the best of both worlds. Food for thought: white flour is the backbone of virtually every baked good you've ever eaten. When cooking with white flour, a baked recipe will usually call for the addition of water, and flour + water = paste. Yup, just like the paste kids use in elementary school. Imagine the sluggishness this "paste" translates to on your digestion. For a healthier middle ground, try cooking with whole wheat flour instead. Whole wheat flour is considered "hard"—it has a much higher protein content than "soft" white flour. Make a pact with yourself to go for whole wheat when making your bread purchases, too.*

Ingredients:

1 tablespoon active dry yeast

2 cups warm water

⅓ cup honey

2 cups whole wheat flour

1 teaspoon salt

⅓ cup vegetable oil

5 cups all-purpose flour

Preparation:

1 Preheat the oven to 375°F.

2 Dissolve the yeast in the warm water. Add the honey, and stir well. Mix in the whole wheat flour, salt, and vegetable oil. Work the all-purpose flour in gradually. Turn the dough out onto a lightly floured surface, and knead for at least 10 to 15 minutes. When the dough is smooth and elastic, place it in a well-oiled bowl.

3 Turn it several times in the bowl to coat the surface of the dough, and cover it with a damp cloth. Let the dough rise in a warm place until doubled in bulk, about 45 minutes. Punch down the dough. Shape into two loaves, and place into two well-greased 9 x 5-inch loaf pans. Bake for 25 to 30 minutes; allow it to rise until the dough is 1 to 1½ inches above the pans.

BALSAMIC CHICKEN PASTA
with FRESH CHEESE

Makes 4 Servings

I really enjoy the combination of protein and dairy, definitely not a kosher option but one that is nutritious and satisfying. Balsamic is one of my favorite flavor enhancers and it provides many health benefits—the Bible even mentions its use as a medicinal tonic. Balsamic vinegar retains many of the nutritional benefits of the grapes from which it is made, such as cancer-fighting polyphenols.

Ingredients:

8 ounces whole wheat linguine

1 red bell pepper, julienned—bursting with vitamins A, C, and K

2 tablespoons balsamic vinegar

3 garlic cloves, minced

½ teaspoon salt

¼ teaspoon pepper

6 tablespoons extra-virgin olive oil—follow the Mediterraneans:
   use it inside and out

1 cup julienned fresh basil leaves

2 cups shredded, cooked chicken

1 cup halved small fresh mozzarella balls

½ cup crumbled soft goat cheese

Preparation:

1 Cook the linguine according to the package directions; drain.

2 Sauté the bell pepper in a small skillet over medium heat until limp, about 12 to 15 minutes.

3 Meanwhile, whisk the vinegar, garlic, salt, and pepper in a small bowl; slowly whisk in the oil. Stir ½ cup of basil into the dressing.

4 Place the pasta, chicken, cooked peppers, mozzarella, goat cheese, and remaining basil in a large bowl. Pour the dressing over the top and toss to coat.

WALNUT-MISO DIP

Makes About 1½ Cups

M iso is an enzymatic, fermented paste made from soybeans that can reduce triglycerides in the blood. It's sweet, savory, and pungent when you eat it by itself, but, when you put it in soup, or mix it into a chip or veggie dip, it's savory and incredibly good for you. One cup of miso soup a day will fight belly fat, too. Miso contains all essential amino acids, making it a complete protein. It helps stimulate the secretion of digestive fluids in the stomach. It restores beneficial probiotics to the intestines. It is also high in antioxidants that protect against free radicals.

Ingredients:

1 cup walnuts, or pecans if you prefer—selenium

3 tablespoons sweet or mellow miso (in the Asian foods aisle)

¾ cup vegetable stock or water

1 to 2 teaspoons rice syrup, optional

Preparation:

1 In an unoiled medium-size skillet, roast the walnuts (or pecans) over medium heat, stirring constantly, for 5 to 7 minutes, or until golden brown and fragrant.

2 Place the roasted walnuts in a blender along with the miso and stock, and blend until smooth. If desired, add rice syrup to taste. Use immediately. Covered and refrigerated, the dip will keep for about 3 days.

TIP: The simple act of drinking a glass of water before each meal is a great weight-loss strategy. It fills your belly with liquid, reducing the amount of space left for food. Your stomach gets full more quickly, sending signals to your brain to "stop eating, you're full."

PRO TIP Get extra benefits from your drinking water by crushing your vitamins and dissolving them in the glass before drinking to make vitamins more bioavailable. Your skin will glow with the benefits.

GREEN BEANS with WALNUTS

*I*n this simple side dish you get the benefits of a very good source of vita-mins, minerals, and plant-derived micronutrients from the beans, and healthy, brain-lubricating fats from walnuts, the "intellectual nut" (observe their kernel's convoluted surface—resembles the brain, no?). Walnuts also help to lower total cholesterol, as well as LDL or "bad cholesterol," and increase HDL or "good cholesterol" levels in the blood.

Ingredients:

3 tablespoons olive oil

½ cup crushed walnuts

1 tablespoon plus ¼ teaspoon truffle sea salt

1 pound green beans, ends trimmed

¼ teaspoon freshly ground black pepper

Preparation:

1 Bring a large pot of water to a boil. Meanwhile, heat the olive oil in a medium skillet over medium heat. Add the walnuts, stir and sear until golden brown, about 3 minutes. Remove from the heat and set aside.

2 Add 1 tablespoon of truffle sea salt to the boiling water, then add the beans and cook until just tender, 4 to 5 minutes; drain.

3 Add the beans, pepper, and the remaining ¼ teaspoon of salt to the skillet and return to medium heat to heat through, 1 to 2 minutes. Use tongs to combine.

MEXICAN QUINOA SALAD

Makes 2 Servings

Quinoa is one of the most protein-rich foods we can eat. It comes from a leafy plant native to South America. It is also a complete protein containing all nine essential amino acids and contains almost twice as much fiber as most other grains. Olé!

Ingredients: Salad

1 cup uncooked red quinoa—superfood

1¾ cups water

1 (14-ounce) can black beans, drained and rinsed—fiber

2 small zucchini or one large, chopped

1 red bell pepper, chopped—superfood

¼ cup finely chopped fresh cilantro

1 cup corn kernels (fresh is best)

1 avocado, chopped into 1-inch pieces

Dressing

4 to 5 tablespoons fresh lime juice (from 2 limes)

¼ cup olive oil

½ teaspoon freshly ground black pepper

½ teaspoon kosher salt

¼ cup finely chopped fresh cilantro

2 garlic cloves, minced

1 teaspoon ground cumin
—works as a weight-loss aid

Preparation: Salad

1 In a medium saucepan, combine the quinoa and water. Bring to a boil and simmer for 15 to 20 minutes.

2 Allow the quinoa to cool for about 5 minutes after cooking. Fluff with a fork. Add the remaining ingredients and toss well.

Dressing

1 Whisk together all the ingredients.

2 Drizzle the dressing over the salad and toss well with additional salt and pepper to taste. Bring the salad to room temperature before serving.

SINFUL SKIN-FUL NACHOS

Makes About 48 Nachos

Here you have my famous nacho recipe that doesn't make your skin feel greasy and your gut feel queasy when you're done eating it. Lots of my celebrity clients adore this one, but probably not as much as I adore them. Sinfully satisfying for the salt craving with lots of beauty benefits built-in, too.

Ingredients:

6 wheat tortillas—rich in selenium

1 tablespoon canola oil—rich in fatty acids

½ cup shredded low-fat cheddar cheese—vitamins A and D and calcium

6 diced black olives—monounsaturated fats and vitamin E

½ tablespoon ground flaxseed powder

3 tablespoons sour cream—lactic acid, a natural exfoliator

Preparation:

1 Preheat the oven to 350°F.

2 Cut each tortilla into eight triangular pieces and place them on a baking sheet. Drizzle them with the canola oil and bake for 10 minutes.

3 When the chips start to get crisp, sprinkle on the cheddar cheese and black olives and put them back in the oven just long enough for the cheese to melt.

4 Mix the flaxseed powder with the sour cream, top each nacho with a dollop of the mixture, and serve.

BEAN and CHEESE
BREAKFAST BURRITO

Makes 1 Serving

*T*his breakfast will keep you powered all the way until lunchtime. Packed with protein and fiber, it's a winning combo that's sure to give you a solid burst of energy in the morning.

Ingredients:

½ cup diced green bell pepper—antioxidant source

1 teaspoon minced jalapeño pepper—a thermogenic food that helps burn away calories

3 egg whites—pure protein, low cholesterol

2 tablespoons shredded cheddar cheese—calcium

¼ cup black beans, if using canned, rinse and drain—fiber

⅓ cup 1-inch chopped, canned green beans, drained

1 small whole wheat tortilla—whole wheat keeps you feeling fuller longer

Salsa or hot sauce, optional

Preparation:

1 Liberally oil a small pan with cooking spray and preheat it over medium heat. Sauté the bell pepper and jalapeño until tender, about 5 minutes.

2 In a small bowl whip together the egg whites. Add the egg whites to the pan and scramble until cooked through. Remove the cooked egg mixture from the heat and mix in the cheese, and black and green beans.

3 Add the mixture to the center of the tortilla. To make a burrito, fold up the bottom of the tortilla (to prevent the filling from spilling out), and then fold over both of the sides. Add a dollop of spicy salsa or hot sauce to give your burrito a kick.

PECORINO and BEAN SALAD

When it's time to spill the beans, you know I will be there with a ready fork and a thoughtful ear. I like pecorino for this salad because it contains an omega-6 polyunsaturated fatty acid, which can actually help fight fat. Say cheese!

Ingredients:

2 tablespoons extra-virgin olive oil

2 cloves garlic, minced

2 teaspoons finely chopped fresh rosemary leaves—dietary fiber, folic acid; can be grown in your kitchen

2 cups shelled edamame beans—star legume of the soy family

1 (15-ounce) can cannellini beans, drained and rinsed—a traditional Italian bean with a nutty flavor

5 ounces pecorino, cut into ½-inch chunks

¼ cup chopped fresh Italian parsley—flavonoids

¼ teaspoon salt

¼ teaspoon finely ground black pepper

Preparation:

1 In a small, nonstick skillet, heat the oil over medium-low heat. Add the garlic and cook until fragrant, but not brown, about 30 seconds. Remove the pan from the heat and stir in the rosemary. Set aside.

2 Combine the edamame beans, cannellini beans, cheese, parsley, salt, and pepper in a serving bowl. Add the garlic mixture and toss well until all the ingredients are coated.

SPAGHETTI SQUASH in
HOMEMADE TOMATO SAUCE

Makes 10 Servings

The whole family will love this dish, especially kids who may be amused by the orange spaghetti in their bowl. In fact, this is a fun dish to make with kids—if you're up for a little splash of tomato sauce here and there. It's always wonderful to see a child's eyes widen with delight when they learn something new about everyday stuff they already know all about (wink, wink). Spaghetti made from a squash? So unique! So healthy! Spaghetti squash is high in manganese, which aids in the production of healthy bones, tissues, and sex hormones. The spaghetti squash variety can be considered a summer or winter squash and is available year-round in most grocery stores; you will need one for this recipe. Now hit the sauce....

Ingredients: Sauce

4 pounds medium-size tomatoes—important source of lycopene,
    a key antioxidant
¼ cup olive oil
1 medium onion, diced
4 to 5 cloves garlic
½ teaspoon salt, plus more, to taste
½ teaspoon red pepper flakes
Fresh oregano, to taste
Fresh basil, to taste
Fresh parsley, to taste

Spaghetti Squash

1 (5-pound) spaghetti squash

Preparation: Sauce

1 Bring a large pot of water to boil. Then, cut a small X on the bottom of each tomato. Place the tomatoes in the boiling water for about 30 seconds, then place in a colander and rinse under cold water, or place in an ice water bath. This cold process is called "shocking" and will maintain the tomato's integrity after having been boiled. Peel the tomatoes; discard the skins.

2 Quarter the tomatoes. Place a bowl under a strainer to reserve the juices. Squeeze the seeds out of the tomatoes over the strainer (this is the messy part). Then coarsely chop the tomatoes.

3 Heat the olive oil in a large pot over medium heat. Cook the diced onions for about 3 to 5 minutes. Add the garlic and cook 2 minutes. Add the tomatoes and bring to a simmer, then lower the heat to medium-low and simmer for about 10 minutes. The tomatoes should be tender at this point. Using a potato masher, gently break up the tomatoes while they are in the pot. Continue to simmer for about 30 to 40 minutes. If needed, add the reserved tomato juice until the sauce reaches the desired consistency.

4 Mix in the seasonings.

Spaghetti Squash

1 Preheat the oven to 400°F.

2 Cut the spaghetti squash in half, lengthwise, and scoop out the seeds. Bake flat-side down on a greased cookie sheet for 35 minutes.

3 After baking the squash, remove it from the oven and scoop the flesh with a large fork (a serving fork, for example). Scrape the long strands of flesh from top to bottom until you've removed enough that you've reached the skin.

4 Add the strands to the pasta sauce.

5 Turn the stove flame to low and heat the sauce with the squash just to warm.

6 Salt and pepper, to taste.

 ## Toning Tomato Mask

Gently mash 1 large tomato in a small bowl. Mix in 2 tablespoons of camu camu extract and 1 small can of tomato paste to act as a binder. Apply to the face and let it sit for 5 to 10 minutes. When your skin feels tingly, wash the mask off.

TOMATO SOUP with RICE and ONIONS

Makes 8 to 10 Servings

T*he soup that eats like a meal, this tangy tummy warmer is rich in vita-mins and minerals.*

Ingredients:

1 large onion, quartered and thinly sliced

½ cup finely chopped celery—hydration

1 medium carrot, sliced—beta-carotine

3 tablespoons butter

8 large tomatoes, peeled, seeded, and chopped

8 cups chicken broth (can replace 1 to 2 cups of broth with V8 drink
  for more added flavor)

3 tablespoons uncooked long-grain rice or rice blend

½ teaspoon salt

⅛ teaspoon dried thyme leaf, or to taste

Freshly ground black pepper, to taste

¼ cup finely chopped fresh parsley

Preparation:

1 In a saucepan, sauté the onion, celery, and carrot in the butter until softened but not browned. Add the tomatoes and a small amount of chicken broth. Simmer for 15 minutes.

2 In a Dutch oven or stockpot, combine the sautéed vegetables, remaining chicken broth, and rice. Season with salt, thyme, and pepper. Simmer 20 to 30 minutes.

3 Serve garnished with parsley.

The Tomato, a Nutrient Powerhouse

Tomatoes are packed with powerful antioxidants like lycopene, which is a great hydrator. Lycopene is said to help protect the skin from age-enhancing UV light from the inside out. Antioxidants are powerful neutralizers of free radicals that damage human cells, causing premature aging. Try to eat one tomato a day. It will help with brightening and hydrating your skin.

BLACK BEAN–OATMEAL BURGERS

<u>Makes 8 Burgers</u>

For something totally different that mimics the experience of burger eating, but with less fat calories and more protein and fiber, try these bean burgers. They are very satisfying and vegan-friendly.

Ingredients:

1 (14.5-ounce) can diced tomatoes, drained well

1 (15-ounce) can black beans, drained well—fiber

1 cup fresh cilantro

2 teaspoons ground cumin—skin-care ingredient

3 cloves garlic, minced—heart healthy

2 green onions, thinly sliced

⅔ cup shredded carrots—vitamin A power food

1¾ cups rolled oats

Preparation:

1 Preheat the oven to 400°F.

2 Add all the ingredients to a food processor and mix well. Form 8 patties and press them flat on a parchment-lined baking sheet.

3 Bake for 20 minutes. Carefully turn over and bake for another 15 minutes. Eat right away or let cool and freeze.

PINTO BEAN–CHIPOTLE TACOS

Makes 2 Tacos

*P*into beans are from Peru. They are an excellent source of fiber and protein. And who doesn't love tacos? And if I may spill the beans here: pin-
tos are fat-free and loaded with vitamins, iron, and several minerals. The
manganese and copper present in the beans are important cofactors of the
oxidative enzyme. This enzyme helps disarm free radicals, which cause
aging. Lots of power in the tiny pinto bean.

Ingredients:

2 medium onions

2 cloves garlic, minced

2 (6-ounce) cans pinto beans, low sodium, rinsed, and drained

¾ cup chicken broth, low sodium (or vegetable)

1½ teaspoons finely minced chipotle chile peppers in adobo
   sauce—a powerful seasoning that adds heat

2 red bell peppers, sliced into thin strips

Salt and pepper, to taste

8 corn tortillas, use lard-free option—niacin

Preparation:

1 Generously coat a medium saucepan with oil spray and heat
  over medium heat.

2 Finely dice ½ of 1 onion and put the diced onion in the
  saucepan along with the garlic. Sauté until the onions are
  tender and translucent, about 5 minutes.

3 Add the beans, broth, and chipotle and bring the mixture to a boil.
  Reduce the heat to medium-low and simmer for 10 to 15 minutes,
  or until most of the liquid has evaporated.

4 While the beans are simmering, generously coat a skillet with
  oil spray and heat over medium heat. Thinly slice the remaining
  1½ onions and add them to the skillet along with the bell peppers.
  Sauté the onions until soft and the peppers until slightly browned,
  about 10 minutes.

5   Using a potato masher, roughly mash the bean mixture (make it as smooth or chunky as you like). Season with salt and pepper, to taste. (If you're using regular canned beans with added salt, you shouldn't need to add any salt to the recipe.)

6   Heat a small skillet over medium heat for warming the tortillas. Place 1 tortilla in the pan and heat for 10 to 15 seconds. Flip the tortilla over and heat for another 10 to 15 seconds, then transfer it to a plate. Repeat with the remaining tortillas.

7   Fill each tortilla with about ¼ cup of the bean mixture. Top with the sautéed peppers and onions and any other preferred toppings.

HEARTY LENTIL SOUP

Makes 4 Servings

Hero Recipe!

For body tone and texture, this very affordable and functional little legume can work wonders. Perhaps you cook with them already, or maybe you are new to these tiny lens-shaped protein pods. In fact, lentils have been a part of the human diet since Neolithic times. They range in color from yellow to orange to red, green, brown, and black. Any color variety, no matter how you cook them, is very good for you. Lentils are high in dietary fiber, folate, and vitamin B_1. Lentils are seeds, not beans, so you don't have to worry about gassy aftermath. They are low in calories and contain virtually no fat. Of all legumes and nuts, lentils contain the third-highest levels of protein. Hands down, they are one of the healthiest foods in the world. This is also a great dish for vegetarians who need new sources for getting protein. Eating lentils helps reduce blood cholesterol because lentils contain high levels of soluble fiber.

Ingredients:

1 large onion, chopped

3 medium carrots, peeled, halved lengthwise, and cut into
 ¼-inch half moons

1 tablespoon extra-virgin olive oil

3 garlic cloves, minced

2 tablespoons tomato paste

1½ cups lentils, picked over and rinsed

½ teaspoon dried thyme

2 (14-ounce) cans reduced-sodium chicken broth—3½ cups

1 tablespoon red wine vinegar—internally healing properties and great
 for a dash of sharp flavor

1½ teaspoons coarse sea salt

¼ teaspoon freshly ground pepper

Tabasco sauce, to taste

Preparation:

1 In a Dutch oven (or other 5-quart pot with lid), cook the onion and carrots in the olive oil, until softened, about 5 minutes. Stir in the garlic, and cook until fragrant, about 30 seconds. Stir in the tomato paste, and cook for 1 minute.

2 Add the lentils, thyme, broth, and 2 cups of water. Bring to a boil; reduce to a simmer. Cover; cook until the lentils are tender, 30 to 45 minutes.

3 Stir in the vinegar, salt, and pepper. Top with Tabasco. Serve immediately.

PANZANELLA
(BREAD and TOMATO SALAD)

Makes 6 Servings

An Italian delight that's just right: this salad's got body, vitamins, and fresh yet complex flavor. Buon Appetito.

Ingredients:

½ cup diced red onion—helps lower blood-sugar levels

4 to 5 medium-size tomatoes, diced

1 cucumber, peeled and diced—hydration and low-cal

2 garlic cloves, chopped

½ teaspoon black pepper

1 tablespoon fresh capers, drained and rinsed—low in fat and calories and
   a relatively good source of fiber and iron

¼ cup chopped parsley

¼ cup chopped fresh basil, or 2 tablespoons chopped fresh thyme

½ head Romaine lettuce (about 3 cups), torn into bite-size pieces—
   enormous nutritional value: protein, calcium, omega-3s, and vitamin C

½ cup crumbled feta cheese—this goat's milk cheese has about 33 percent
   fewer calories than most cheeses

2 teaspoons Dijon mustard

2 tablespoons red or rice wine vinegar

3 tablespoons olive oil

2 cups whole-grain bakery-style bread, cut into ½-inch cubes—you may
   use stale bread if you have it, that's the classic method!

Preparation:

Mix all the ingredients together (except the bread). Spoon onto bread chunks and serve immediately.

HEIRLOOM TOMATO SALAD with POMEGRANATE DRIZZLE

This is one of my go-to, antioxidant-rich, sweet/savory light salads I can consume multiple servings of and still never feel stuffed or bloated. Just totally satisfied.

Ingredients:

3 tablespoons extra-virgin olive oil

2 tablespoons pomegranate molasses*

2 pounds mixed heirloom tomatoes, sliced ¼-inch thick
   —extra flavorful and lycopene loaded

Sea salt, such as Maldon*, to taste

½ teaspoon pepper

2 tablespoons fresh oregano leaves

You can find pomegranate molasses and Maldon sea salt at well-stocked grocery stores and gourmet shops, or go online to search and purchase these key pantry items.

Preparation:

1 Whisk together the oil and molasses.

2 Arrange the tomatoes on a platter. Drizzle with the molasses dressing.

3 Sprinkle with salt and pepper and scatter oregano on top.

STRAWBERRY-BUCKWHEAT PANCAKES

Makes 3 to 4 Servings

A gluten-free alternative to regular or whole wheat pancakes, buck-wheat pancakes rise up nice and fluffy and have a warm, earthy, rich flavor. Diets that contain buckwheat have been linked to a lowered risk of high cholesterol and high blood pressure. Strawberries are sweet, delicious, and amazing for their antioxidants and vitamins that create healthy-looking skin. Buckwheat offers a rich supply of flavonoids, particularly rutin. Flavonoids are lipid-lowering phytonutrients; in conjunction with vitamin C antioxidants, you've got strong skin-aging weapons with this recipe. Buckwheat also contains almost 86 milligrams of magnesium in a one-cup serving. Magnesium relaxes blood vessels, improving blood flow and nutrient delivery while lowering blood pressure—the perfect combination for a healthy cardiovascular system.

Ingredients:

Canola oil for coating the pan—omega-3s

1½ cups buckwheat flour

3 tablespoons Truvia Baking Blend

½ teaspoon salt

1 teaspoon baking soda

1 teaspoon ground flaxseed

3 tablespoons salted butter, melted, plus more, for topping

1 tablespoon honey

1 egg

2 cups buttermilk—probiotic for pearlescent skin

1 small crate strawberries—about 4 ounces

Maple syrup, for topping

Preparation:

1 Heat a well-seasoned griddle, cast-iron skillet, or a stick-free pan on medium heat. The pan or griddle should be oiled with canola oil and ready for the batter as soon as it is mixed.

2 Whisk together the dry ingredients—the flour, Truvia Baking Blend, salt, baking soda, and flaxseed—in a large bowl. Pour the melted butter and honey over the dry ingredients and start stirring. Beat the egg with a fork and stir it into half of the buttermilk. Add the buttermilk mixture to the dry ingredients, then slowly add in the rest of the buttermilk as needed to get to the right consistency for your batter (you may not need all of the buttermilk, depending on what type of buttermilk you are using and the brand of flour). Stir only until everything is combined. Do not overmix. A few lumps are fine.

3 Ladle the batter onto the hot surface to the desired size, about 4 to 5 inches wide. (A ¼-cup measure will ladle about a 4-inch pancake.) Reduce the heat to medium-low. Allow the pancake to cook for 2 to 3 minutes on this first side. Watch for bubbles on the surface of the pancake. When air bubbles start to rise to the surface at the center of the pancake, flip the pancake. Cook for another 1 to 2 minutes, or until nicely browned.

4 Keep your pancakes warm on a rack in an oven set on warm, or stack them on a plate and cover with a towel as you make more. Spread more oil on the pan as needed between batches of pancakes. Serve with butter, maple syrup, and strawberries.

CAMU CAMU POPOVERS

SERVINGS 6

These are the classic popovers with an anti-aging twist. Camu camu is a superfruit bursting with ultrahydrating vitamin C.

Ingredients:

Flour, sugar, or Parmesan cheese for dusting muffin tray

3 large eggs

1 cup milk

3 tablespoons melted butter

1 cup flour

½ teaspoon salt

1 tablespoon Truvia

1 teaspoon camu camu powder

Preparation:

1 Preheat the oven to 400°F. Grease each cup on a muffin tray and lightly dust with flour, sugar, or Parmesan cheese, your choice.

2 Have all ingredients at room temperature. In a blender, beat the eggs, add the milk and melted butter, and slowly blend in the flour, salt, Truvia, and, lastly, the camu camu powder.

3 Fill each popover (muffin) cup ¾ full and bake for approximately 50 minutes.

4 Remove and serve immediately. For a drier popover, prick the top of the popover with a toothpick in the last five minutes of baking.

BERRY BLAST PIZZA

Makes 4 Servings

*T*he go-to food to help reduce loose skin and increase muscle tone is . . . *BERRIES! Here's the simple takeaway: eat sweet berries, and do well by your body. Blueberries, strawberries, blackberries, black raspberries, red raspberries, cranberries, and purple grapes (with skin) are rich in antioxidant compounds called anthocyanins, which help the skin with elasticity and full-body glow. Berries are a marvelous natural sugar treat.*

Ingredients:

4 fajita-size (6-inch) flour tortillas
⅓ cup seedless raspberry all-fruit jam
1 cup part-skim ricotta cheese
1 cup raspberries—low-cal superfruit
1 cup blackberries—low-cal superfruit
1 cup hulled and halved, or quartered if large, strawberries—low-cal superfruit
1 cup blueberries—low-cal superfruit

Preparation:

1 Preheat the oven to 350°F. Place the tortillas on a baking sheet and top each with a tablespoon of jam, spreading it almost to the edge. Bake until the tortilla is crisp, about 10 minutes. Remove and cool to room temperature.

2 Spoon ¼ cup of ricotta over each tortilla, spreading it almost to the edge. Divide the berries among the tortillas, making alternating rows of raspberries, blackberries, strawberries, and blueberries. Brush the tops with the remaining jam. Serve immediately, cutting into wedges like a pizza.

Blackberries and raspberries are technically not considered botanical berries despite their antioxidants and the suffix "berrie" in their name. They fall into a subset category called aggregate fruits, which means they are a fruit that develops from the merger of several varieties that were separate in a single flower. The category of "simple fruits" includes those that develop from one berry, which is good for your health and your skin.

STRAWBERRY-KIWI CUPCAKES

*H*ealthy and delightful. The New Zealanders had it right when they assumed the nickname "Kiwi." As for the fuzzy kiwifruit, it's the national fruit of China and is rich in vitamins C, K, and E. Paired with strawberries, vanilla, and almond milk you get a cupcake with nutrition—and body benefits, too.

Ingredients:

1 cup butter

1½ cups Truvia Baking Blend

2 eggs—protein brain-boosters

2 teaspoons vanilla

4 cups flour

4 teaspoons baking powder

1 teaspoon salt

1 cup almond milk—light, nutty, crisp—magnesium, potassium

1½ cups diced strawberries

2 kiwis, peeled and diced

Preparation:

1 Preheat the oven to 400°F. In a mixing bowl, cream together the butter and Truvia Baking Blend until fluffy.

2 Mix in the eggs and vanilla.

3 In a small bowl, combine the flour, baking powder, and salt. Stir for a minute with a whisk or fork. Alternately add the flour mixture and milk into the mixing bowl. Stir just until combined, being careful not to overmix.

4 Carefully fold in the strawberries and kiwis.

5 Scoop the batter into greased muffin tins and bake for about 15 to 20 minutes, until golden brown and cooked through.

Frosting:

2 (8-ounce) packages cream cheese, softened

½ cup butter, softened

1 teaspoon vanilla extract

1 tablespoon red palm oil (turns frosting pink and powers it up!)

Beat the cream cheese and butter until combined. Add the vanilla and the red palm oil and mix well.

GRILLED SALMON with FRUIT SALSA

Makes 4 Servings

Hero Recipe!

A tropical topping on a cold-water fish dish makes for a delicious pairing of sweet and savory—one of my favorite combinations. Salmon is a great source for heart-healthy omega-3s. Anytime you can get another omega in your body, the better. Add this to antioxidant-rich fruit and you've got an anti-aging body benefit recipe.

Ingredients: Fruit Salsa (Makes 2 Cups)

¾ cup diced pineapple

¾ cup diced mango—tropical superfruit rich in prebiotic dietary fiber

½ cup diced strawberries

¼ cup small diced red onion

1 jalapeño stemmed, seeded, and finely chopped

2 tablespoons chopped fresh mint leaves—can help eliminate toxins from the body when included in the diet regularly

2 tablespoons orange juice

1 tablespoon fresh lime juice

¼ teaspoon iodized salt

1 teaspoon honey

Salmon

4 (6-ounce) salmon filets, skin on

4 teaspoons olive oil, divided

2 teaspoons Zatarain's Creole seasoning

Preparation: Fruit Salsa

In a medium porcelain or glass bowl, combine all the ingredients and stir to blend. Cover with plastic wrap and allow the salsa to marinate for 30 minutes before serving with the fish.

Salmon

1 Preheat the grill to medium.

2 Brush both sides of the salmon with the olive oil. Season the salmon on both sides with the Creole seasoning. Place the fish on the grill skin-side down, and cook for about 3 minutes, then turn the fish 45 degrees and cook for an additional 3 minutes. Turn the fish over and cook for an additional 2 minutes, or until cooked through to the desired degree of doneness.

3 Remove the fish from the grill and serve with the fruit salsa spooned on top. Serve immediately.

 Honey-Mango Facial

Honey retains moisture so your skin feels hydrated and fresh all day.
It also absorbs impurities from the pores in the skin, making it a very effective chemical-free remedy to help clear skin blemishes like acne and pimples.
You will need 4 tablespoons of finely chopped mango pulp, 1 to 2 teaspoons of honey, and 1½ tablespoons of almond oil. Combine all the ingredients in a bowl and mix well. Using a clean foundation brush (or your fingertips), apply to a clean face and neck. Leave the mask on for 15 to 20 minutes. Rinse off thoroughly with lukewarm water. Good for all skin types.

LIME-CHICKEN SATAY with TROPICAL SALSA

Makes 4 Servings

*T*he addition of lime to these skewers adds a bright taste. The abundance of lime in this recipe is beneficial for skin. Internally and externally, lime rejuvenates skin, keeps it shining, protects it from infections, and can even reduce body odor due to its large amounts of vitamin C and flavonoids. Flavonoids are beneficial to skin due to their antioxidant activity.

Ingredients:

4 (4-ounce) boneless, skinless chicken breasts

3 tablespoons lime marmalade

1 teaspoon white wine vinegar

½ teaspoon finely grated lime zest

1 tablespoon freshly squeezed lime juice

Salt and freshly ground black pepper, to taste

Preparation:

1 Slice the chicken breasts into long, thin strips, and thread onto bamboo skewers that have been soaked in water for 30 minutes.

2 Preheat the broiler. Mix together the lime marmalade, vinegar, lime zest, and lime juice in a small bowl. Season, to taste, with salt and pepper.

3 Arrange the chicken skewers on the rack in a broiler pan and coat generously with the lime marmalade mixture. Cook under the broiler for 5 minutes. Turn the chicken over, brush with the mixture again and broil for another 4 to 5 minutes, until the chicken is no longer pink inside.

TROPICAL SALSA

A simple healthy salsa that's ready to eat. Use it as a dip for chips, or enjoy it right out of the bowl.

Ingredients:

4 medium tomatoes, cored, seeds removed, chopped

2 medium cloves garlic, finely minced

2 to 3 tablespoons finely chopped sweet onion

1 to 2 tablespoons minced jalapeño

2 heaping tablespoons finely chopped cilantro

2 tablespoons fresh lime juice—vitamin-C antioxidant power

1 mango, peeled and chopped

½ peeled, cored, and chopped fresh pineapple

½ cup chopped strawberries

Preparation:

In a bowl, combine all the ingredients and stir to blend.

 Lime Body Scrub

When applied directly on the skin, the acids in lime scrub away dead cells, help reduce rashes, and make for a refreshing bath if lime juice or oil is mixed into your bathing water. Slice open a lime and rub it on the skin. Wash off and follow with a rich shea butter moisturizer.

BROCCOLI, SPINACH, and CHEESE QUICHE

Makes 8 to 10 Servings

Quiche is a bona fide comfort food ideal for breakfast, lunch, or dinner. You can even eat quiche as a cold leftover with a dash of Tabasco sauce. Broccoli, surprisingly, has more vitamin C than oranges. It is a good source of fiber and plant omega-3s. Broccoli is also high in folic acid, which is of particular importance for pregnant women.

Ingredients:

1 prepared 12-inch piecrust or homemade piecrust
1 tablespoon vegetable oil
1 cup chopped onions
1 cup shredded cheddar cheese—calcium
1½ cups frozen broccoli, defrosted
⅓ cup spinach
¾ cup half-and-half
2 eggs
½ teaspoon salt
Pinch of pepper

Preparation:

1 Preheat the oven to 400°F. Place a cookie sheet in the middle of the oven. Poke the piecrust with a fork a few times. Place the pie pan on the cookie sheet and bake for 5 minutes in the preheated oven to set the crust.

2 While the crust is baking, heat the oil in a small skillet over medium high heat. Add the onions and sauté them for 2 to 3 minutes, until lightly browned.

3 Remove the crust from the oven. Sprinkle shredded cheese over the bottom of the piecrust, then add the onions. Place the broccoli florets around the outside of the crust with the stems facing the center. Next lay the spinach circling in toward the center of the crust. Finally, add a couple of small florets in the center.

4   In a medium-size bowl, combine the half-and-half, eggs, and salt. Mix until smooth, then pour into the piecrust. Return the pan to the oven.

5   Bake for 10 minutes, then turn the temperature down to 350°F and continue cooking until a knife inserted into the custard comes out clean, about 50 minutes.

6   Remove and let the quiche stand for a few minutes before cutting.

TIP: Diets high in cruciferous veggies help reduce risk of memory loss and cancer. Try broccoli, Brussels sprouts, cabbage, kale, spinach, and Swiss chard. Open your hand, stack your green three layers high, then eat. These veggies also contain lutein, which helps protect the skin from sun-induced inflammation and wrinkles.

TOFU SPINACH DIP

Makes 4 Servings

*T*ofu *is nutritious enough to replace meat—not that I recommend that you do—but if you are vegetarian, tofu's got you covered. Tofu (and soy) have flavonoids that are great for skin and have been found to be a great source of calcium and vitamin E as well. This recipe also calls for water chestnuts, an aquatic veggie that is crunchy and nutty. Water chestnuts add fiber and potassium, are low in sodium, and go beyond Asian-food dishes.*

Ingredients:

2 (8-ounce) packages extra- or medium-firm tofu—protein-packed soy

1 cup fat-free mayonnaise

1 lemon, juiced

3 to 6 cloves of garlic, to taste

1 packet Lipton's onion soup mix, dry

2 teaspoons dried parsley

½ teaspoon dried thyme

2 tablespoons white chickpea miso—live lactobacilli enhance the body's ability to extract nutrients from food

1 tablespoon dried dill weed

1 teaspoon dried basil—anti-inflammatory properties

Ground pepper, to taste

10 ounces frozen spinach, thawed and drained

1 can water chestnuts, drained and chopped

4 green onions, sliced—chromium, sulfur, and B_6 for heart health

Sourdough or olive bread

Preparation:

1 Blend all the ingredients *except* the spinach, water chestnuts, green onions, and bread in a food processor until smooth. Scrape down occasionally.

2 Add the spinach to the processor after the other ingredients are smooth and pulse until the spinach is chopped and well blended. Put the mixture into a bowl and stir in the water chestnuts and green onions. Chill overnight. Serve with sourdough or olive bread.

SPICY CURRY DIP

Makes 4 Servings

This one's egg- and dairy-free, with a bite of Indian spice. Makes for a unique, low-calorie hors d'oeuvre.

Ingredients:

1 cup well drained, soft tofu

3 cloves garlic, crushed

1 teaspoon cayenne powder—can help clear clogged arteries

2 tablespoons curry powder—skin superfood with antibacterial properties

½ teaspoon salt

Juice of 1 lemon

Preparation:

In a blender, blend all the ingredients until smooth and creamy. Serve with veggies cut into sticks, or crackers.

BOK CHOY SALAD

Get back your salad days! Bok choy is Chinese for "white vegetable," a leafy green and white-stem veggie that's loaded with vitamins A and C, which are good for your skin. This type of Chinese cabbage is commonly found in markets around the world. The combination of ingredients in this salad lends itself to a decidedly "Asian" flavor—tangy, bright, and gently spiced. It's a scrumptious salad, very low in fat and yet extremely satisfying. I served it in a massive cut-crystal punch bowl at a pool party, and it was completely devoured.

Ingredients:

2 to 3 heads bok choy   1 bunch scallions—low-calorie antioxidant

Noodle Mixture

1 to 2 package(s) soba noodles   ¼ cup sliced almonds

¼ cup raw sesame seeds—rich in mono-   1 teaspoon garlic salt
  unsaturated fatty acid and oleic acid

Salad Dressing

¼ cup grapeseed oil—love this, so healthy—great for skin and hair glow

2 tablespoons toasted sesame oil

¼ cup rice or cider vinegar

Generous squeeze of agave syrup or raw sugar

2 tablespoons soy sauce—digestive tract benefits

¼ cup fresh ginger

1 to 2 cloves garlic

Preparation:

1 Wash and cut the white and green parts of bok choy into bite-size pieces. Dry the bok choy well using a salad spinner. Wash and slice the scallions into thin rings (white and green)

2 Crush the soba noodles by hand. Heat the oil over medium heat to brown the noodles, sesame seeds, and sliced almonds. Season with garlic salt. Set aside.

3 Combine the salad dressing ingredients in a food processor. Toss and mix the 3 mixtures together just before serving. The three mixtures can be made ahead and stored in separate containers.

How Low Can You Go?

Chapter 5

Just because the lower regions of the body are mostly covered by clothing doesn't mean they're unimportant, or unseen. If you like warm-weather climates and summertime (I think we all do), sooner or later, your raised, red, or irritated skin; dry feet, cracked heels, yellowing or striating toenails; and orange peel–like skin will be revealed! Even dry hands (from washing hundreds of times a day with kids, for example) can be a prime target for age obviousness. Brown spots on the hands are another age giveaway.

Think about it: You aspire to protect your face and nourish your body but neglect SPF on the hands? And those fabulous, long-lasting color gel manicures where you put your hands in the UV light box? This is the same type of UV light from a tanning bed—akin to setting the Benjamin Button–button full speed ahead! A friend of mine who partakes in these long-lasting color gel manicures coats her hands in sunblock first and proceeds to wear fingerless gloves during the UV light-box time—a bit obsessive, or smart protection? You be the judge.

In this chapter, you will learn how to boost your beautiful skin and body, and target common challenges. The journey toward luminous beauty runs neck and neck with the long and winding road toward aging. But here's some basic drugstore wisdom: You can stave off looking old. We all eventually suffer the damaging effects of gravity, repeated sun exposure, and countless treats and cocktails that were less than salubrious. Damaging. Dam-aging! So, what can you do to undermine these challenges without the aid of a scalpel? Sure, a new pair of hot boots might make you feel like a million bucks, as could a trip to the barber for an old-fashioned hot shave with an old-fashioned straight-edge razor and some neighborhood gossip. But why not start by simply feeding your body what it craves?

TOP 5 Hero Foods for Loving Thy Body

Peppers (sweet and/or hot, red, green, chiles)—contain thermogenic capsaicin to help burn fat.

Olive Oil—contains a series of compounds beneficial to most functions of the human body.

Papaya—rich in antioxidants.

Mushrooms—help protect the immune system.

Honey—offers incredible antiseptic, antioxidant, and cleansing properties for body and health.

CHICKEN SAUTÉ with BELL- and CHILE-PEPPER KICK

Makes 4 Servings

Hero Recipe!

Lots of healthy things are happening in this dish. A great source of protein among slenderizing veggies, such as tricolored bell peppers, rich in anti-oxidant carotenoids, heart-healthy garlic, and vitamin C–rich chile pepper.

Ingredients:

¼ cup grapeseed oil, divided
4 skinless, boneless chicken breast halves, cut into strips
Salt and pepper, to taste
1 red bell pepper, thinly sliced
1 yellow bell pepper, thinly sliced
1 orange bell pepper, thinly sliced
1 medium onion, thinly sliced
1 medium-size red chile pepper, chopped fine
4 cloves garlic, finely chopped
1 tablespoon dried basil
¼ cup balsamic vinegar, divided

Preparation:

1 Heat 2 tablespoons of grapeseed oil in a large skillet over medium-high heat. Place the chicken in the skillet, season with salt and pepper, and brown on both sides. Remove from the heat, and set aside.

2 Heat the remaining oil in the skillet over medium heat, and stir in the red bell pepper, yellow bell pepper, orange bell pepper, onion, and chile pepper. Cook for about 5 minutes, until tender. Mix in the garlic, and cook and stir for about 1 minute. Mix in the basil and 2 tablespoons of balsamic vinegar.

3 Return the chicken to the skillet. Reduce the heat to low, cover, and simmer 20 minutes, or until the chicken is no longer pink and the juices run clear. Stir in the remaining balsamic vinegar just before serving.

BAKED TILAPIA
with BELL PEPPERS

<u>Makes 4 Servings</u>

The most commonly found bell peppers are green, red, orange, or yellow, but purple, blue, brown, and white bell peppers are out there, too. Green bell peppers are more bitter than the other colors, giving them a slightly sharper flavor that's more acidic. When cooked, the acid is absorbed by the juices and the fish. Go with the color you like.

TIP: If you buy fresh tilapia fillets, avoid musky scents. If you buy frozen tilapia, carefully check the fish when thawed and discard it if it feels mushy, or if its smell makes your nose crinkle. The fish should also have moist, shiny, and tightly adhering scales.

Ingredients:

¾ cup extra-virgin olive oil, divided

4 tablespoons tomato paste—lycopene to protect cells from free radicals

1 teaspoon garlic powder

1 teaspoon dried oregano

¼ teaspoon salt

⅛ teaspoon ground black pepper

4 (4-ounce) tilapia fillets—a fab, flab-fighting fish!

2 bell peppers, sliced into thin rounds

1 onion, sliced into thin rounds—flavonoids

4 tablespoons butter

Preparation:

1 Preheat the oven to 350°F.

2 Use roughly ¼ cup of olive oil to grease the bottom of a baking dish.

3 Mix the remaining ½ cup of olive oil with the tomato paste, garlic powder, oregano, salt, and pepper in a small bowl.

4 Place the tilapia fillets in a large baking dish with the skin-side up.

5 Use a spatula to spread the olive oil mixture over the fish.

6 Surround the tilapia fillets with bell peppers and onion.

7 Place the dish in the preheated oven and bake until the tilapia fillets can be easily flaked with a fork. This will normally take around 15 minutes.

8 Remove the dish from the oven and place 1 tablespoon of butter on top of each tilapia fillet. Set the oven to broil; broil the fish until the butter melts and becomes slightly brown, about 4 to 7 minutes.

GRILLED FISH TACOS with RADISH-CABBAGE SLAW

Makes 4 Servings

Radishes are low in digestible carbohydrates, high in roughage, and contain a lot of water. They are a wee bit sharp in flavor—kind of like a potato-onion sans onion breath—and a good dietary option for those determined to lose weight. I think they balance and work nicely in this tangy slaw.

Ingredients:

1 garlic clove, minced

½ teaspoon sea salt

¼ cup finely chopped fresh cilantro, plus leaves for serving

1 teaspoon chipotle chile powder

1 teaspoon dried oregano

1 lime, zested and juiced, plus 4 lime wedges for serving

1 lemon, zested and juiced, plus 4 lemon wedges for serving

1 teaspoon grapeseed oil

4 (5-ounce) red snapper fillets, skin on—selenium, vitamin A, omega-3s

8 radishes, julienned—rich in folic acid

6 ounces green cabbage, finely shredded (about 2 cups)

2 scallions, julienned

1 firm avocado, peeled and pitted

½ tablespoon honey

8 (4-inch) flour tortillas

Preparation:

1 Mash the garlic and salt into a fine paste and transfer to a bowl. Stir in the cilantro, chipotle powder, oregano, lime and lemon zest, and grapeseed oil. Cut 2 slashes in the skin of each fish fillet. Flip, and rub half the spice mixture onto the fish; reserve the remaining half.

2 Heat a grill pan over medium-high heat. Grill the fish, skin-side up first for about 4 minutes. Flip once, until cooked through, about another 4 minutes.

3 Remove the skin from the fish, and discard. Flake the fish into large pieces, discarding any bones. Combine the fish with the remaining spice mixture and toss with 1 teaspoon lime juice and 1 teaspoon lemon juice.

4 Toss the radishes, cabbage, and scallions in a bowl. Mash the avocado in a separate bowl; stir in ½ tablespoon of lime juice, ½ tablespoon of lemon juice, and ½ tablespoon of honey.

5 Heat the tortillas in a skillet over high heat, and amass onto a plate.

6 Spread mashed avocado onto each tortilla. Top with the fish, slaw, and cilantro leaves. Fold the tortillas over the filling, and serve with lime and lemon wedges.

CAST-IRON SKILLET JALAPEÑO MAC and CHEESE

Makes 4 Servings

Thisis my personal favorite dish. It satisfies that comfort food craving while offering health benefits, too. Cooking with cast iron is simply an option, but I find that the heat retention works nicely for this bubbly mac and cheese, and that it settles best when cooked this way. Jalapeños, a type of pepper, promote circulation. Ever notice how eating hot, hot peppers clears out your sinuses and makes your eyes water? That's the heat of capsaicin working its magic (see Hot, Hot, Hot! on page 159). This recipe requires a 10¼-inch cast-iron skillet; I know it's heavy, but I like cooking with cast iron because even the tiny flecks of iron the food may pick up from the skillet are good for you.

Ingredients:

8 ounces whole wheat elbow macaroni—fiber; digestion

3 tablespoons butter

¼ cup chopped onion

3 tablespoons flour

½ teaspoon salt

⅛ teaspoon black pepper

1 cup heavy cream—lactic acid

½ cup white wine

2½ cups extra sharp grated cheddar cheese

2 fresh jalapeños, muddled (mashed/mixed together)—combat nasal congestion

Drizzle of truffle oil—omega-3s; anti-inflammatory and anti-aging; great for overall health and vigor

Preparation:

1 Cook the macaroni in boiling salted water according to the box directions. Drain. Set aside.

2 Meanwhile, in a 10¼-inch cast-iron skillet over a large burner, melt the butter, add the onion, and sauté until tender. Stir in the flour,

salt, and pepper. Slowly add the cream and wine. Cook over low heat, stirring until thickened. Add the macaroni. Stir in the cheese until melted. Top with the jalapeños and a drizzle of truffle oil. (Take care not to touch your eyes or broken skin with errant jalapeño juice.)

3 Cook in the oven at 350°F until the top is browned and bubbly, about 20 minutes.

Hot, Hot, Hot!

Hot peppers—caliente, tasty, and high performance—the hotter the chile pepper, the greater the benefit. Habañero, jalapeño, red chile peppers, chipotle, cayenne, hot sauce . . . they all contain capsaicin. Capsaicin has potent antibacterial and anti-inflammatory properties that can help fight and even prevent chronic sinus infections or sinusitis by stimulating secretions that help clear mucus from your nose. Hot peppers are a good source of vitamins A, C, and E, potassium, and folic acid, with no carbohydrates. If you have a sensitive stomach, hot peppers may not be well tolerated by your system. That burn in your mouth you get from a good hot pepper will contribute to a rise in body temperature, energy expenditure, and appetite control.

 ## Chile Pepper Wake-Up Call

Use hot chile pepper on the skin to help with circulation—great for dimply skin on the legs, tummy, and the rest of the body. A quick, targeted body serum would be to muddle chile pepper or a chile paste with grapeseed oil and rub it on the skin before a hot shower. When you feel the tingle, that's when you should wash it off. If you want to reap the daily benefits of this bump-busting serum, use an empty plastic cosmetic jar or lotion bottle (you can buy at the 99-cent store), fill it with shea butter, and add the serum to the shea butter. Two tablespoons serum added to about 8 ounces of lotion should suffice. By the way, the 99-cent store is the go-to place for cheapie versions of shea butter, cosmetic jars of all sizes, hair bands, mixing spoons, paint brushes you can get a few uses out of for makeup application, and so forth. Why not start your own home-spa beauty bar? Experiment and have fun with it.

BACON-JALAPEÑO
CORNBREAD

Makes 4 Servings

W*hen I was growing up, we called this the BJC. If your mom made it, you were a BMOC (big man on campus). It is so savory and delicious, and I used to run home after basketball to devour entire portions of it. I don't do too much devouring anymore, nor do I shoot many hoops these days, but I still love this cornbread and hope you will, too. It's an easy preparation and you get body benefits from the jalapeño, cornmeal, milk, and garlic.*

Ingredients:

1 cup cornmeal—rich in antioxidants

1 cup flour

2½ cups milk

1 onion, grated—disease fighter!

3½ teaspoons baking powder

½ cup vegetable oil—can increase HDL [good] cholesterol

3 eggs, beaten

2 tablespoons Truvia Baking Blend

1 small can of cream corn (or 3 ears of fresh corn cut and scraped)

½ cup chopped jalapeño peppers

1½ cups grated cheese, your choice

¼ pound bacon, fried crisp, dried on paper towels, and crumbled

¼ cup chopped canned pimento

1 to 2 cloves garlic, chopped or crushed

Preparation:

Preheat the oven to 400°F. Mix all the ingredients together and bake in a large greased rectangle baking pan for 35 minutes.

VEGETARIAN CHILI

Makes 4 Servings

Because they're high in soluble fiber, beans help fight cholesterol, and for those who don't eat meat, this vegetarian chili dish gets a good hearty flavor that is robust and satisfying. I like the black bean and chickpea combination, but use your favorites to satisfy your taste buds and those of your family.

Ingredients:

1 tablespoon olive oil

1 large onion, coarsely chopped

3 cloves garlic, minced

1 pound butternut squash, peeled, seeded, and cut into ½-inch chunks
   —full of antioxidants, minerals, and vitamins

1 red bell pepper, ribs and seeds removed, cut into 1-inch chunks

¼ teaspoon chipotle chile powder—rich in minerals, iron, niacin, thiamin, magnesium, and riboflavin

Coarse salt and ground pepper, to taste

1 (14.5-ounce) can stewed tomatoes in juice

1 (19-ounce) can chickpeas, drained and rinsed—protein

1 (19-ounce) can black beans, drained and rinsed—fiber

1 (8-ounce) can button mushrooms, drained

½ cup chopped cilantro, divided—essential oils

Lime wedges, for serving

Preparation:

1 In a Dutch oven or 5-quart saucepan with a lid, heat the oil over medium heat. Add the onion and garlic and cook, stirring occasionally, until tender, for 5 to 7 minutes. Add the squash, bell pepper, and chile powder; season with salt and pepper and cook, stirring, for 1 minute. Add ½ cup water. Cover and simmer until the vegetables are crisp-tender, about 7 minutes.

2 Stir in the tomatoes and their juice, breaking them up with a spoon; add the chickpeas, black beans, mushrooms, ¼ cup cilantro, and ½ cup water. Bring to a boil. Reduce to a simmer, partially cover, and cook until lightly thickened, about 20 minutes.

3 Season with salt and pepper. Stir in the remaining cilantro and spoon into serving bowls. Serve with lime wedges.

PAPAYA CARROT SALAD

<u>Makes 1 Serving</u>

If this fruit reminds you of the tropics and you can envision yourself lying on a sandy beach with an exotic cocktail in hand, then eat it quick! You need fruit like papaya to help target bumpy skin and improve skin elasticity, which should be of interest to you if you are, well, lying on the beach. Talk about an anti-aging superfood! This antioxidant is one of nature's wonders, improving digestion and arthritis, among many other bodily challenges. Papaya will help you fight off cold and flu viruses and help keep you healthy through the winter due to its high content of flavonoids, vitamins, and minerals. The ripe fruit is usually eaten raw and has a wonderfully soft, butter-like consistency and a sugary musky taste.

Ingredients:

1 large carrot

1 papaya

¼ cup extra-virgin olive oil

1 tablespoon honey

2 red chiles, chopped (adds heat and flavor, contains high amounts of vitamin C and carotene)

1 lime, juiced, seeds removed

⅛ teaspoon freshly ground black pepper

⅛ teaspoon iodized salt (the iodine in salt has healing properties)

Preparation:

1 Dice the carrot into bite-size pieces. Pit the papaya and slice it lengthwise into ½-inch-thick pieces. Place all the pieces in a small bowl.

2 In a separate bowl, combine the remaining ingredients and stir. Spoon this dressing over the carrot and papaya. Serve immediately.

Pumpkin-Papaya Revitalizing Facial

To gently remove dead skin cells and firm tired flesh, a mud scrub with powerful fruit enzymes will revitalize skin. Mix pumpkin and papaya with Kaolin clay, or with any clay or "mud" mask you may have in your medicine cabinet. Apply to clean skin; leave on until dry. Remove by flushing the skin with cold water, then moisturize. This is also a great treatment for legs to tighten up tired-looking skin. When done, slather a rich cream onto legs.

 ## Honey, Your Hands

Honey is a natural moisturizer and ambrosia of so many uses. For this skin-smoothing treatment you will need to sacrifice one pair of socks that you do not mind discarding after use. Using a paintbrush or a synthetic fiber makeup brush, dip the brush into a jar of raw honey and generously paint a layer of it, about ¼-inch thick, onto one hand and then cover it like a mitt with one of the socks. Then, with your honey-mitten hand, do the same for your other hand. Leave on for 30 minutes and then rinse off thoroughly. Your hands reveal your age, sometimes even more so than your face, so smooth out and soften your hands to reverse the clock.

Bad Breath? Take Papaya.

Notice any changes in your breath lately? With aging comes the onset of pungent smells from deep within. You may be an A+ toothbrusher, flosser, and mouthwasher, but yet you still find you have the occasional bad breath. If you have this problem, look no further than the papaya. The fruit, as well as the other parts of the papaya tree, contain papain, an enzyme that helps digest proteins. If you're not getting them directly from the fruit, store-bought, chewable, papaya enzyme supplements are widely available. They will help break down certain types of food in the stomach, which benefits digestive health. You can also get the benefits from papaya teas, cooked papaya in stews and curries, papaya juice, and dried papaya fruit. Choose the form that best fits your diet and lifestyle.

TANGY TIGHTER-TUMMY SALAD

Makes 4 Servings

*O*kay . . . *nothing you can eat makes a tummy tighter, but this is a tasty salad you can enjoy to keep it from becoming "fluffier." In my opinion, this dish is like a light and refreshing version of coleslaw. Everyone who has tasted it at my house loves it. The capsaicin in the chile pepper can reduce hunger and increase energy expenditure, in turn burning calories. Water-rich grapefruit hydrates your body and makes you feel fuller, jicama [hih-ka-muh] is low in carbs and high in fiber. Pistachios are one of the lowest fat, highest fiber nuts around. So dig in.*

Ingredients: Vinaigrette

1 small, thin Serrano chile, diced—vitamin C

1 large garlic clove, chopped

3 tablespoons fresh lime juice

1 tablespoon dark brown sugar

1½ tablespoons Asian fish sauce (a flavor booster that can be used in place of salt, commonly found in the Asian foods aisle in supermarkets)

Salad

3 grapefruits, peeled and segmented

1 medium carrot, peeled and shredded

⅓ cup cilantro leaves, divided, leaving 2 tablespoons as garnish

¾ pound jicama, peeled and shredded—low-cal root veggie, vitamin C, fiber

2 tablespoons crushed, roasted pistachios, as garnish

Preparation:

1 In a small bowl, whisk together the vinaigrette ingredients.

2 In a large serving bowl, toss together the salad ingredients. Lightly coat with the vinaigrette. Scatter the pistachios on top and garnish with 2 tablespoons of remaining cilantro leaves.

CHICKEN ENCHILADAS VERDES

<u>Makes 8 Servings</u>

Make a great dinner tonight that tastes decadent and is good for you, too. Sour cream gives your skin health-promoting lactic acid, and skinless chicken breasts are a supreme, low-fat protein. These enchiladas are made with a fresh green salsa, just like you would find in a Mexican restaurant. Your dining companions will be verde with envy over this recipe.

Ingredients:

1½ pounds bone-in chicken breast halves, skin removed
½ medium white onion, halved crosswise
1 whole clove garlic
½ teaspoon coarse salt
2 cups loosely packed fresh cilantro
1½ pounds tomatillos, husked and rinsed
1 jalapeño chile
1 poblano chile
8 (6-inch) corn tortillas
2 ounces reduced-fat Monterey Jack cheese, grated (about 1 cup)
½ cup sour cream, thinned with 2 tablespoons water

Preparation:

1 Place the chicken, ½ of the onion, the garlic, and ¼ teaspoon of salt in a medium saucepan. Add enough water to cover by at least 1 inch. Bring to a boil, and then reduce the heat.

2 Simmer until the chicken is cooked through, 18 to 22 minutes. Reserve ¾ cup of the cooking liquid; set aside.

3 Let the chicken cool on a plate. When cool enough to handle, shred (discard bones).

4 Coarsely chop ½ cup of cilantro, and toss with the chicken.

5 Preheat the broiler, with the rack about 6 inches from the heat source. Broil the tomatillos and chiles on a rimmed baking sheet, rotating them as they blacken, 10 to 12 minutes. Let cool. Remove the

blackened skins, stems, ribs, and seeds (optional) from the mixture. Reduce the oven temperature to 375°F.

6 Coarsely purée the tomatillos and the chile mixture in a blender with the remaining ¼ teaspoon of salt, the remaining 1½ cups of cilantro, and the reserved ¾ cup of cooking liquid. Transfer the salsa to a large bowl.

7 Using tongs, toast the tortillas over an open flame of a gas stove, 5 to 10 seconds per side. (Or heat the tortillas in a skillet over high heat.)

8 Dip 1 tortilla into the salsa to coat lightly. Place ⅓ cup of the chicken mixture on half of the tortilla. Sprinkle 2 tablespoons of cheese on top, and roll up. Place it seam-side down in a 9 x 13-inch baking dish. Repeat to make more enchiladas, lining them up snugly in the dish. Spoon the remaining salsa on top, and bake until heated through, about 20 minutes.

9 Slice the remaining ½ onion, and scatter over the top; drizzle with sour cream.

RICOTTA and SPINACH STUFFED NOODLES

Makes 6 to 8 Servings

Hero Recipe!

Part-skim ricotta keeps calories at bay; spinach and bulgur deliver anti-oxidants and fiber. The complex carbs in pasta boost serotonin, the mood-stabilizing neurochemical, which is what makes pasta a comfort food.

Ingredients:

1 (28-ounce) can whole tomatoes

2 tablespoons good olive oil

1 onion, finely diced

2 cloves garlic, minced

Coarse salt and ground black pepper

¾ cup boiling water

½ cup bulgur—a natural weight-loss food high in fiber and protein

2 packages whole-grain lasagna noodles

1 pound spinach, stems removed—vitamin A promotes healthy skin

1 (15-ounce) container part-skim ricotta cheese

1 egg, beaten—protein

¼ cup freshly grated Parmesan

Preparation:

1 Pulse the tomatoes and their juices in a food processor until smooth.

2 Heat the oil in a medium pan over medium heat. Sauté the onion and garlic until tender, about 7 minutes. Add the tomatoes and cook, stirring until slightly thickened, about 20 minutes. Season with salt and pepper. Let the sauce cool.

3 Heat the oven to 350°F. Pour boiling water over bulgur, cover, and let stand until it's soft and the water is absorbed, about 30 minutes.

4 Cook the lasagna noodles in a large pot of salted boiling water. Drain, remove, and lay out flat; let cool.

5 Steam the spinach, covered, over medium heat, stirring occasionally, until tender. Gently squeeze out the excess moisture, coarsely chop, and add to the bulgur. Stir in the ricotta. Season with salt and pepper. Stir in the egg.

6 Coat the bottom of a 9 x 13-inch casserole dish with 1 cup of sauce. Spoon the filling into the noodles, wrap, and arrange in the pan with the seam-side down. Add the remaining sauce, cover with foil, and bake until bubbling, about 40 minutes. Sprinkle with Parmesan before serving.

TBG SHELLS

Makes 3 to 4 Servings

*T*hese *tomato-basil-garlic shells are so good. There's nothing quite as comforting as sitting down to a steaming hot bowl of plentiful pasta, and sharing kind conversation with a friend. Add a bottle of wine to the mix and you're totally in the zone. Serve this dish to an acquaintance and upgrade to BFF. Beauty-boosting ingredients such as garlic and cherry tomatoes in these TBGs will TCB (take care of business), and leave your tummy happy.*

Ingredients:

⅓ cup extra-virgin olive oil

2 large garlic cloves, finely chopped

About ¾ teaspoon kosher salt

1¼ pounds (1 quart) small cherry and teardrop tomatoes—lycopene

¾ pound medium seashell pasta (if you can find them in whole wheat, even better)

½ cup shaved Parmesan cheese—high in calcium

½ cup thinly sliced fresh basil leaves—helps fight the common cold

Preparation:

1 Combine the oil, garlic, and salt in a large bowl. Chop 1 cup of the tomatoes and add to the bowl. Cut the remaining tomatoes in half and stir into the mixture; let stand about 30 minutes, stirring occasionally.

2 Cook the pasta as the package directs in a large pot of salted boiling water.

3 Drain the pasta, saving 1 cup of water. Toss the pasta with the tomato mixture, then add the cheese and all but 1 tablespoon of basil. Mix in a little pasta water if needed for a looser texture. Sprinkle the remaining basil on top and season with salt.

TIP: To slough off dead skin on elbows and legs, mix kosher salt with olive oil and scrub on skin for an exfoliation treatment. Or oil up first, then put salt in a saltshaker and sprinkle it on before scrubbing. It feels like light magical rain and leaves skin remarkably soft.

VA-VA'S PUMPKIN PANCAKES

*P*ower to the pumpkin. Kids love pumpkins for the obvious reason: pumpkins = Halloween = candy! But you can leverage this gourdlike squash in so many other ways. Pumpkins contain high levels of beta-carotene, in the form of vitamin A. A single-cup serving of pumpkin or other winter squash has 145 percent of a child's daily requirement for vitamin A. Pumpkin also boasts vitamin C, potassium, fiber, manganese, folate, omega-3 fatty acids, thiamin, copper, tryptophan, and B-complex vitamins. If you like pancakes, these are your healthy option. Va-Va would be proud.

Ingredients: Pancakes

1 cup whole wheat pancake mix

1 cup filtered water

⅓ cup canned pumpkin—excellent source of carotenes

½ teaspoon cinnamon

¼ teaspoon ground ginger

1 teaspoon probiotics powder—alkalizing, provides true energy to
   a depleted body

Syrup

5 tablespoons toasted pumpkin seeds

1 cup simple syrup flavored with vanilla extract—maple syrup counteracts
   the pumpkin taste so stick with simple syrup

Preparation: Pancakes

1 In a medium bowl, whisk the pancake mix, water, pumpkin,
   cinnamon, and ginger into a lumpy consistency.

2 Spray the griddle with nonstick spray and warm over medium heat.

3 To form a pancake, spoon roughly 2 tablespoons of batter onto the
   griddle. Cook until bubbling, flip, and cook for 2 additional minutes.

4 Plate the pancakes, sprinkle on probiotics powder, then top
   with syrup.

Syrup

1 Preheat the oven to 350°F. Roast the seeds for 5 minutes on a foil-lined baking sheet.

2 Remove the seeds from the oven and combine with the syrup in the bowl.

 ### Anti-Aging and Clarifying Pumpkin-Lettuce Facial

Pumpkin is excellent for skin clarity. Rubbed on the face or body, or ingested, pumpkin enzymes work wonders on the skin. If you can eat them and rub them on, you get the power of two, the best for inside-out health and beauty. Try this anti-aging and clarifying facial:

You will need some iceberg lettuce leaves and a small can each of condensed milk and pumpkin mix. Wash and dry the lettuce and place in the freezer for a few minutes until the leaves are ice cold. Start your facial by cleansing the skin with a gentle exfoliator. Then layer on your face the condensed milk—a thick lactic acid penetrator. Follow by layering on the canned pumpkin. Go thick. Next, press the chilled lettuce leaves onto your face until your face is covered. Leave on for 15 to 30 minutes, or as long as you can stand it. Remove the lettuce when through, and rinse your face with warm water.

TIP: I use and believe in glycolic acids for exfoliation, but I prefer lactic acid. Glycolic acid is highly volatile when you work with it directly on bare skin. It is best used in a cream or lotion base that acts as a cushion between the acid actives and bare skin. Lactic acid is just as effective, but it's derived from milk acid so it's gentler even when used in higher concentrations than glycolic acids.

Secrets from Va-Va

Use a dab of olive oil to massage toenails, cuticles, nail corners, and nail beds. This will not only soften skin and cuticle brittleness but will release tension and sensations of tightness from your toes, and subsequently, your feet.

Care for Bruised, Neglected, or Tired Tootsies

- **Athlete's foot.** Soak feet in an Epsom salt bath to help relieve the symptoms of athlete's foot.
- **Splinters.** Soak affected skin area in an Epsom salt bath to draw out the splinter.
- **Toenail fungus.** Soak your affected toes in hot water mixed with a handful of Epsom salt three times a day.
- **Sprains and bruises.** Add 2 cups of Epsom salt crystals to a warm bath and soak to reduce the pain and swelling of sprains and bruises and replenish the body's magnesium levels.
- **Dry skin patches.** To gently scrub away dry skin patches, mix 2 cups of Epsom salt with ¼ cup of petroleum jelly and a few drops of lavender essential oil. This will exfoliate beautifully. Alternately, mix Epsom salt with olive oil for a targeted exfoliation.
- Finally, after showering, you can massage handfuls of Epsom salt over wet skin to exfoliate your body. It's the same treatment many upscale spas use. It feels crumbly, tingly, and effective!

Notes on Nails and Pretty Feet

For callused feet. Soak your feet in warm water with 1 Alka Seltzer tab for 10 minutes. Then use a foot file, pumice stone, or exfoliating scrub to remove calluses.

Fungus among us? Cuticles keep out germs, so treat them well. Tell your nail technician not to push back or cut your cuticles during a pedicure. This lowers your risk for infection. In between visits, never tear or pick your cuticles. Over time, you can end up with deeply ridged, unsightly nail beds. Soften ragged cuticles by rubbing in moisturizer as often as you can remember to. If you notice that your cuticles are red or irritated, see your doctor.

At-Home Pedi Tips

Before you polish your nails, gently clean underneath them with a manicure stick. Wrap a small tear of tissue around the point like they do at the salon. To trim your toenails in between pedicures, cut them straight across to help prevent ingrown toenails. This also keeps them strong.

Pedicures are fabulous for a host of reasons. Who doesn't love a good pedicure? They make feet look pretty, dainty, and sexy with open-toe shoes, and they take care of the rough bits we can't get close enough to examine ourselves. But here's the thing, nails need to breathe and have moisture, and polish acts as a barrier. It may be hard to commit to this, but try skipping the nail polish for a week or longer each month and enjoy the low-maintenance look. Do it in the wintertime. Let your toenails see the light of day and you will notice that the yellowing starts to fade.

Pedi Rules

Don't shave your legs before a pedicure. Your pedicurist has seen it all before, so your hairy gams are no surprise, and not at all out of the ordinary. Bacteria have a better chance of getting into your body through tiny nicks or cuts on freshly shaved legs. And despite the thorough cleaning nail salons are supposed to do in-between customers, certain kinds of bacteria live in tap water and can thrive in a dirty footbath. Wait until after your pedi to shave. You can also take your own tools to a nail salon, and many salons sell tool kits, too. Germs can linger on salon implements that aren't cleaned, such as emery boards. If you choose to use the salon's tools, they should be heat sterilized, soaked in clear antibacterial solution, or come prepackaged. Ask for a new tool if one falls on the floor during your appointment. Never feel intimidated to politely ask for what you want during your treatment. You are paying for a service and you deserve to experience it the way you wish. No one should be hampering your ME time! If they massage too hard, let it be known. Tip well and you will get an A+ treatment time and time again.

SHRIMP and SPINACH
SHIITAKE MUSHROOM RISOTTO

Makes 4 Servings

*P*erhaps you have bigger fish to fry, but know this: Shrimp are the sexy fish. Why? Because they have virtually no fat and are packed with protein, making them the ultimate weight-management food, and, although they don't travel well due to the need for refrigeration, shrimp are a great healthy snack, raw or cooked. This recipe also calls for shiitakes—the gourmet super mushroom! They have a meaty flavor that is delicious and contain an active component called lentinan, which strengthens and stimulates immune response, helping to clear out infection and disease. The shiitake mushroom also contains a good supply of long-chain sugars called polysaccharides, which provide a long-burning fuel source. They're an excellent source of vitamin D, too, and they can reduce cholesterol. Risotto is a rich multi-ingredient dish that is based around rice as its main starch.*

Ingredients:

3¾ cups reduced-sodium chicken broth

1½ cups chopped fresh shiitake mushrooms (smoky flavor)
   —immune system support

1 small onion, chopped

1 tablespoon butter

3 garlic cloves, minced

1 cup uncooked arborio rice—healthy grain

1 (6-ounce) package fresh baby spinach, coarsely chopped

1 pound cooked medium shrimp, peeled and deveined

½ cup shredded Parmesan cheese

¼ teaspoon pepper

Preparation:

1 In a small saucepan, heat the broth and keep it warm.

2 In a large nonstick skillet, sauté the mushrooms and onion in butter until tender, about 3 minutes. Add the garlic; cook for 1 minute longer. Add the rice; cook and stir for 2 to 3 minutes. Carefully stir

in 1 cup of the heated broth. Cook and stir until all of the liquid is absorbed.

3 Add the remaining broth, ½ cup at a time, stirring constantly. Allow the liquid to absorb between additions. Cook just until the risotto mixture you have created is creamy/loose in the skillet and the rice is almost tender, about 20 minutes.

4 Add the spinach, shrimp, cheese, and pepper; cook and stir until the spinach is wilted and the shrimp are heated through.

CHICKEN POTPIE SQUARES
with MUSHROOMS

Makes 6 Servings

*I*f you've got leftover chicken (or turkey), making a potpie is a great way to finish it off and turn it into a different meal. Potpie is a satisfying dish that incorporates protein, starch, vegetables, and spices in every forkful. I ate many of them when I traveled through London. To knock off some time, in this recipe you will be baking the entire pie in one dish, rather than breaking it out into mini-pie tins. You can square off your portions to the desired size after.

Ingredients: Filling

1½ pounds boneless, skinless chicken breasts

½ cup baby carrots

2 cups chicken broth

½ cup dry white wine

2 teaspoons fresh (or ¾ teaspoon dried) thyme leaves

12 ounces fresh mushrooms, halved or quartered if large—powerful nutrients; low-cal, fat-free, cholesterol-free, very low in sodium

½ cup sliced red bell pepper

2 tablespoons vegetable oil

2 garlic cloves, peeled and finely minced

3 tablespoons flour

2 tablespoons cream or half-and-half, optional

Salt and pepper, to taste

¼ cup grated Parmesan cheese

Topping

One 8 x 12-inch rectangle of prepared puff pastry dough, thawed*

1 egg white mixed with 1 teaspoon water in a bowl

2 tablespoons grated Parmesan cheese

1 teaspoon fresh (or ¼ teaspoon dried) thyme

*Note: For tender, flaky crusts, choose heat-resistant glass pie plates or aluminum pie pans with a dull finish. Shiny pie pans are not recommended because they reflect heat, causing a soggy bottom crust.

Preparation:

1 Combine the chicken, carrots, broth, wine, and thyme in a saucepan and simmer for approximately 8 to 10 minutes until the chicken is cooked through. Transfer the chicken and carrots to a plate. When they are cool enough to handle, tear the chicken into pieces. Reserve the broth for later use in this recipe.

2 In a large frying pan, sauté the mushrooms and bell pepper in the oil on medium-high heat, stirring often, until lightly browned. Lower the heat to medium, add the garlic and flour, stir in well until no flour lumps remain, and sauté for an additional minute. Add the cooked chicken and carrots.

3 Gradually add the reserved broth/wine mixture and optional cream, stirring continuously. Simmer for 5 to 10 minutes until the sauce has thickened. Add salt and pepper, to taste. Spoon the mixture into an 8 x 12-inch glass or ceramic baking dish and sprinkle with Parmesan.

4 Place the puff pastry dough on a work surface lightly dusted with flour. Cut the dough into 12 pieces. Brush the top surface of the dough with the egg white/water mix and sprinkle with Parmesan and thyme. Lay the cut dough on top of the chicken in the baking dish.

5 Bake at 400°F for 15 to 20 minutes until the pastry is cooked through and browned.

CRUNCHY CHICKEN TENDERS
with PROBIOTIC DRESSING

Makes 4 Servings

*T*his dish is full of surprises. You get the WOW taste factor of your Sunday football hot wings, but with lean protein breast meat instead of fatty wing meat. The herb-buttermilk dressing has a probiotics base. Probiotics are my all-time favorite beautifiers. They are the major leaguers for boosting beauty. They are "the good bacteria" already alive and thriving in the digestive system. You can treat and even prevent some illnesses with foods and supplements containing certain kinds of live bacteria. Probiotics powder is available inexpensively; it is tasteless and dissolves nicely. You literally can sprinkle it on most any kind of food, or swirl it into dip or dressing, as we do below. Everyone gets the health benefits.

Ingredients: Chicken

1 cup buttermilk
1 tablespoon Dijon mustard
½ teaspoon kosher salt
¼ teaspoon cayenne pepper
2 cups whole wheat breadcrumbs
2 pounds boneless, skinless chicken breast, pounded to even thickness
    and cut into strips
Olive oil, for drizzling

Dressing

⅓ cup buttermilk
3 tablespoons 2 percent Greek yogurt
1 tablespoon minced chives
1 teaspoon probiotic powder
¼ teaspoon kosher salt
1 tablespoon crumbled blue cheese, optional

For Serving

4 stalks celery, cut into sticks
2 romaine hearts, quartered
Hot sauce, to taste

Preparation: Chicken

1 Heat the oven to 400°F. Line a baking sheet with tin foil and spray with nonstick spray.

2 Combine the buttermilk, mustard, salt, and cayenne in a glass or porcelain dish. Place the breadcrumbs in a bowl or spread on a dish. Dip the chicken in the buttermilk mixture, then transfer to the bowl or dish with breadcrumbs, pressing to coat. Place the coated chicken on a baking sheet and drizzle with oil. Bake until the chicken is golden and cooked through, about 16 minutes. Season with salt.

Dressing

For dressing, combine the buttermilk, yogurt, chives, probiotics powder, and salt in a bowl. Add the blue cheese, if desired.

To serve

Serve the chicken with dressing, celery, romaine hearts, and hot sauce.

Eating Probiotics to Beat Inflamed Skin

My good friend's daughter has had eczema since birth. At its worst it was bumpy, bleeding, and staining sheets—and ferociously itchy. After rounds at dermatologists, allergists, and pharmacists, what proved to be the most healing for her was eating probiotic-rich foods. This included basic Kefir yogurt with active live cultures (in all kinds of yummy berry flavors), organic soy yogurt (chocolate is her fave), buttermilk pancakes (a Sunday morning ritual), and daily probiotic powder with two billion cells per serving swirled into her morning milk. The skin-smoothing effects were undeniable, which is why probiotics work for anti-aging. Infuse your daily diet with them: Eat foods that are rich in probiotics and take them in capsule, powder, or tablet form, whichever you prefer. Ingesting probiotics to flush out toxins will help the circulatory system, too.

Nighttime Probiotics for Glowing Skin

Nighttime beauty trick: Take 1 probiotic capsule, gently open the casing, and tap the powder into a dollop of your PM moisturizer. Swirl it into the moisturizer and apply to your face as usual. It may feel pasty; this is normal. The mixture will feel slightly granular, which is why this is best for nighttime treatment. In the morning your skin will glow, and glowing skin is going to be your new normal.

 Home-Spa Treatments for Glowy Nails

1. Soak your nails in a bowl of warm almond oil or olive oil for half an hour daily. Don't wash your fingers but gently massage the oil into your fingernails. Practice this on a daily basis to cure brittle nails, and enhance shine.
2. Apply a mixture of honey and lemon to your fingernails and toenails. Massage this mixture into the nail and do not wash it off if you can manage it.
3. Apply a mixture of a vitamin E capsule and ¼ teaspoon warm olive oil to strengthen brittle nails, and enhance shine.
4. Prepare a scrub to harden nails by mixing a teaspoon of honey, a tablespoon each of olive oil and castor oil, and ½ cup shelled, ground walnuts. Apply this paste to the hands, fingernails, toenails, and feet, and gently scrub them. You may want to eat it—but rinse it off with lukewarm water instead. Repeat twice a week.
5. Before going out, apply a thick layer of milk cream or petroleum jelly to your hands and fingernails and slip on cotton gloves to keep them hypermoisturized.

TIP: Nail ridges may indicate a lack of protein, iron, or calcium. Enrich your diet with those nutrients; otherwise, take silica supplements or get silica from foods such as alfalfa, asparagus, bell peppers, cabbage, corn, cucumbers, flaxseeds, mustard greens, oats, olives, radishes, rice, soybeans, and white onions.

TIP: A warm olive oil soak for 10 to 15 minutes a day for a month, then twice a week thereafter, will help brittle nails. Also, smooth on a generous amount of olive oil to hands before bed; massage hands and rub in well. Put on white cotton gloves, or clinical gloves if you have them, and go to sleep. Your hands will be softer and smoother in the morning, and your nails will be nourished. Follow up with cuticle cream and your weak, thin nails are a goner.

Damaged Nails?
Protein and Biotin to the Rescue!

Fingernails that flake or peel easily are commonly caused by a lack of the protein keratin. Keratin deficiency can also result from crash dieting or other sudden dietary changes. A protein-rich diet can reverse the damage, as can taking a daily supplement of biotin, a B vitamin. Other causes of soft or brittle nails include the chemicals in acetone (nail polish remover) and methyl acrylate (acrylic nails), which are used during manicures and pedicures.

FYI: Nude nails are the new black; let them breathe.

 ## All-Over Body Beauty Bath

If you want help with bumpy, orange peel–like skin, try this Alka Seltzer/oatmeal/honey/milk bath. Run a hot bath; place 2 Alka Seltzer tablets, a bottle of carbonated water, and ½ gallon of milk into the tub. Swirl it around with your hand. Next, add 1 cup of dry oatmeal and ½ cup of honey and get in. The heat of the bath opens your pores; the carbonation of the water makes the active ingredients more effective. Slather the bath mixture on your body (picture yourself in ancient Greece!), and rub it into your skin from head to toe. The Alka Seltzer in the warm lactic acid bath will deeply hydrate, smooth, tone, brighten, and lighten your skin. The oatmeal serves as a natural exfoliant, and the honey is a natural skin conditioner. Add a shea or cocoa butter moisturizer after you towel off and your skin will feel silky and soft.

Living the Sweet Life

Chapter 6

You don't have to give up dessert when you're eating smart. You just have to eat smart(er) desserts. To deprive yourself of sweets is akin to being on a beach without SPF—an outdated and painful notion. For me, the situation always arises when my goal of sticking to a dessert-free eating plan gets outdone by my sweet tooth; yes, the sweets always triumph, and I'm okay with that because I've learned how to eat the right kinds of desserts. But the question remains, how do we satisfy the sweet tooth without the guilt and total lack of nutrition? By now, I know you can help answer that question: add in beauty boosters!

Here's where you get to let loose—just a bit—and have fun experimenting with a something-for-everyone array of dessert recipes that are sweet and satisfying. Any of these desserts are appropriate as a cap to a dinner party, or to eat casually at home after a weekday meal. I think these options have all the right stuff, but there's no sugarcoating the facts: You should enjoy in moderation. And to be sure we're on the same page here, my friend, remember that just because you get a beauty boon doesn't mean you can overindulge. The recipes in this chapter aren't a solution to low-cal dessert consumption, but what you do get are the tools to enjoy savvy desserts with *superfood ingredients* and hopefully a guilt-free good time. We don't want to live life prohibitively, but we want to make smart choices that maximize the goodness God gave us and revel in the delights that come with it.

TOP 5 Hero Foods for Sweet-Tooth Savvy

Dark chocolate—more antioxidant-rich than milk chocolate.

Green tea—antioxidants and steady energy.

Almond milk—more beneficial and nutritious than ordinary dairy milk, due to the fact that it contains more nutrients and it has not been subjected to the same processing.

Fresh cream—lactic acid is good for the complexion.

Goji berries—superfruit antioxidant.

DARK CHOCOLATE, SEA SALT, and AVOCADO COOKIES

Makes About 2 Dozen Cookies

*S*kin-healing ingredients in a decadent dessert are the way to go if you're going to go for it. I love these cookies; they are so innovative and really taste great. Cookies are great for a lunchbag, after-school treat, or weekend snack with a cup of green tea. This recipe is a cool teaching tool for kids, too, showing them how to substitute healthy ingredients for the not-so-healthy ones—and still get full flavor. Eating small amounts of chocolate may boost physical endurance, too. A 5-gram piece of dark chocolate—roughly the size of two postage stamps—is the optimal daily dosage.

Ingredients:

2¾ cups all-purpose flour

1 teaspoon baking soda

1 teaspoon coarse sea salt

1 teaspoon vanilla

5 tablespoons butter

½ medium ripe Hass avocado (about 5 ounces, peeled, pitted, and mashed)—great for skin glow and digestion

1 cup light brown sugar

¾ cup Truvia Baking Blend

2 large eggs

1 (12-ounce) package dark chocolate chips—polyphenols

1½ cups chopped pecans—protein

Preparation:

1 Preheat the oven to 350°F.

2 Mix all the ingredients, except the chocolate chips and pecans, in a large bowl, stirring continuously until smooth.

3 Fold in the chocolate chips and pecans to the mixture.

4 Using a small retractable ice cream scooper or spoon, scoop out ½-inch cookie rounds and drop onto an ungreased cookie sheet.

5 Bake for 8 minutes or until golden brown on the edges.
   Note: cook time can vary slightly by the pan you use, so for the
   first batch set a timer for 8 minutes to start and add more time in
   2 minute increments until the cookies appear to have a golden
   brown outer edge.

6 Allow to cool, and enjoy.

PRO TIP

A sugar scrub of ½ teaspoon of baking soda mixed with raw brown or white sugar will open up pores, help clear skin imperfections, and mattify. Moisten fingers and hands and then rub it on face, décolleté, and neck.

Dark chocolate has several health benefits. The darker the chocolate, the better it is. This is because cacao (the main ingredient in chocolate) contains isoflavanoids, polyphenols, and cacao bioferments, all of which raise antioxidant levels in your body. (Note: Halloween-type milk chocolates—you know the ones—are manufactured and contain processing ingredients and *less* healthful benefits.) If you need to answer to a chocolate fix, go for a bar that's 60 to 90 percent cacao; you'll see the percentage on the packaging. The best kind of chocolate has a high flavanol content and should be at least 60 percent cacao. It's slightly less sweet but is rich and deeply satisfying, even if you take a bite of it plain. (I love 90 percent because it's slightly sweeter.) Dark chocolate helps skin stay hydrated and protects skin from sun damage, and, contrary to popular belief, it does not cause acne. (Indulgently consumed *commercial* chocolates, however, may clog pores due to an abundance of oils, sugars, and other binders of the non-natural variety.) All the more reason to get your delight from pure dark chocolate.

MATCHA GREEN TEA
and CHOCOLATE SWIRL CAKE

<u>Makes 10 Servings</u>

Matcha [mAA-cha] is a tea indigenous to Japan that's very rich in nutrients, antioxidants, and chlorophyll. One glass of matcha is the equivalent of 10 glasses of green tea in terms of nutritional value and antioxidant content! When drinking matcha, whole tea leaves are consumed (not just the steeped liquid, as with other teas), providing 4 to 6 hours of mild, steady energy. Matcha is both a stimulant and a relaxant, perfect for focusing on work, exercise, or play.

Ingredients:

Oil to grease the pan

2 cups all-purpose flour

1 tablespoon baking powder

½ teaspoon salt

4 large eggs

1 cup granulated sugar

1 cup milk—vitamin D

1 cup vegetable oil

1 teaspoon vanilla extract

2 tablespoons unsweetened cocoa powder

1½ tablespoons matcha green tea powder

Preparation:

1 Preheat the oven to 350°F. Grease the bottom of a 10-inch round pan with oil.

2 Stir the flour, baking powder, and salt in a bowl.

3 In a large mixing bowl, mix the eggs and sugar until smooth and light colored, about 2 minutes on high speed with a hand mixer. Add the milk and oil, and mix for another minute. Add in the flour mixture and mix just until blended. The batter will be of pouring consistency but not thin.

4 Stir in the vanilla.

5 Divide the batter evenly into two bowls. Add the cocoa powder to one bowl and mix until blended. Add the green tea powder to the other bowl of batter and mix until blended.

6 To assemble the cake: Using two ¼-size measuring cups, pour a cupful of the white cake batter onto the center of the pan. Then, pour a cupful of the chocolate batter directly on top at the center of the cupful of white cake batter. You will be creating a "tree-ring" pattern as you pour one cup of mix onto the next cup of mix, making the rings spread outward. Repeat until all the batter has been poured into the pan.

7 Bake the cake until a knife inserted at the center comes out clean, approximately 50 minutes. Transfer to a rack and allow to cool. When you cut a slice you will see the alternating color effect in cross-section!

GREEN TEA (or MATCHA) POUND CAKE

Makes 6 Servings

This lovely cake is worthy of your mother-in-law. With only about 4 grams of fat per slice, this special pound cake offers great flavor plus a touch of medicinal green tea. Enjoy it as an afternoon snack with a cup of soothing hot green tea to double your antioxidant gain.

Ingredients:

¾ cup cake flour
¾ cup whole wheat pastry flour, or white for more traditional cake
1½ teaspoons baking powder
1 teaspoon baking soda
¼ teaspoon kosher salt
¼ cup margarine, trans-fat free, reduced-fat, soft tub
¼ cup brown sugar
2 egg whites—low cholesterol, high protein
1 cup buttermilk
2 teaspoons matcha, dissolved in 1 tablespoon hot water
1 teaspoon vanilla extract
1 large Madagascar vanilla bean pod, extracted

Preparation:

1. Preheat the oven to 350°F. Coat a 1-pound loaf pan with cooking oil spray.

2. In a medium bowl, combine the cake flour, pastry flour, baking powder, baking soda, and salt.

3. In a large bowl, beat the soft tub spread and brown sugar with an electric mixer on medium speed until fluffy. Add the egg whites and mix well. Mix in the buttermilk, green tea powder, vanilla, and vanilla bean pod extract.

4. On low speed, mix in the flour mixture until just combined. Do not overmix.

5. Bake for 30 to 35 minutes, or until the top begins to brown and a toothpick comes out clean when inserted in the middle of the cake. Transfer to a wire rack and let cool for 5 minutes. Remove the cake from the pan and cool completely.

GREEN TEA and CHOCOLATE CHEESECAKE

Makes 2 (5-inch) Round Cheesecakes

I would seriously open up an umbrella-topped street stand just to sell these special cheesecakes. Not only do they look exotic, but the taste is outstanding, and, of course, they have beauty-procuring bennies.

Ingredients: Crust

½ cup chocolate wafer crumbs

2 teaspoons Truvia Baking Blend

1½ tablespoons unsalted butter, melted

Filling

5 ounces whipping cream

6 ounces cream cheese

⅓ cup Truvia Baking Blend

3½ ounces almond milk

¾ teaspoon matcha green tea powder

1 teaspoon powdered gelatin, or pectin

Preparation: Crust

1 Preheat the oven to 325°F. Butter the bottom of two (5-inch) round springform pans.

2 Combine the chocolate wafer crumbs, Truvia Baking Blend, and melted butter in a medium bowl until well combined and crumbly. Press firmly into the bottom of the pans with your fingers.

3 Bake in the oven for about 10 minutes. Let cool on a wire rack while you make the filling.

Filling

1 Whip the cream in a stand mixer with the whisk attachment until soft peaks form. Set the cream aside.

2 In a clean mixer bowl, beat the cream cheese until soft and creamy (do not overbeat and liquefy it). Add the Truvia Baking Blend and beat to combine.

3 Heat the almond milk in the microwave in a heatproof cup until almost hot (not boiling). Add in the matcha powder and whisk until combined and there are no lumps.

4 Dissolve the gelatin (or pectin) in about 2 tablespoons of water. Note: Make sure gelatin is liquid or it will not blend smoothly with the cheesecake. If the gelatin is solid, heat in a microwave for 10 seconds at a time until liquid.

5 Add the almond milk to the cream cheese and mix until combined.

6 Fold in the whipped cream gently with a rubber spatula until combined.

7 Add the gelatin to the cheesecake mixture and fold until combined.

8 Pour the cheesecake mixture into the prepared pans. Refrigerate for at least 1 hour until set. Coat the sides in more chocolate crumbs after you unmold the cheesecakes for added *oomph*.

No Wiggle Anti-Aging Gelatin Serum

You will need 1 tablespoon of unflavored, powdered gelatin, 1 tablespoon of water, and 1 or 2 drops of olive oil. Scoop out a tablespoon of the powdered gelatin and mix it with the water and olive oil to create a paste. Gently rub a pearl-size amount of the mixture in your palms and then press the viscous mixture onto your face and neck. Use this in addition to—or in place of—your current anti-aging serum, or use at night as an intensive weekly anti-aging serum. Gelatin is derived from collagen, which is the protein that gives skin elasticity, and the olive oil is ultramoisturizing.

YUMMY NO-BAKE CAROB BARS

Makes About 10 Bars

These are one of my unique treats that are "safe" to have around the kitchen when impulse-snacking hits. With this bake-free recipe, you can whip up tasty carob bars that are full of minerals and proteins for increased health value. Although eaten in ancient Egypt, carob was most popular in the 1970s, and I'm all about bringing it back. There's even a parable in the Jewish Talmud that features carob.

Carob is mildly sweet, a good substitute for chocolate, and can be used to make cakes, cookies, candy, pudding, icing, bread, beverages, shakes, ice cream, muffins, fudge, and brownies. Carob contains as much vitamin B_1 as asparagus or strawberries; as much niacin as lentils or peas; and more vitamin A than eggplant and asparagus. It also contains vitamin B_2, calcium, magnesium, potassium, iron, manganese, chromium, copper, and nickel. It is a good source of fiber. Compared to chocolate, it's three times richer in calcium, has one-third less calories, less fat, and is caffeine-free, but it is also a taste preference and lacks the antioxidants found in dark chocolate.

Ingredients:

2 cups carob chips
½ cup pure maple syrup
2 tablespoons whole milk—vitamin D
4 tablespoons butter
3 cups oatmeal—low-cal, high fiber
½ cup chopped walnuts

Preparation:

1 Grease an 8 x 8-inch glass cake pan with butter. In a saucepan (a double boiler is best), melt together the carob chips, syrup, milk, and butter slowly.

2 Put the oatmeal in a large mixing bowl. When the wet ingredients are melted and stirred together, add the mix to the oats. Then add the nuts. Mix well.

3 Press the mixture into a greased pan. Cut into squares while still warm. Cover with plastic wrap and refrigerate until firm.

CHILLED CAROB CREAM PIE

Makes 12 Servings

*A*nother great tasting dessert from the carob camp with the power of honey, gelatin, and vanilla, too. I love anything that's creamy; I should've worked in a dairy!

Ingredients:

1 large pie shell

6 tablespoons carob powder

8 ounces cream cheese

6 tablespoons honey

1 cup half-and-half—lactic acid

1 tablespoon vanilla

¼ cup cold water

1 package of gelatin

Preparation:

1 Blend everything together except the water and gelatin.

2 Prepare the gelatin according to instructions, then add it into the blended mixture, along with a ¼ cup cold water, and blend well.

3 Pour the mixture into the pie shell. Chill until set.

TIP: Honey is more than a sweetener to squeeze into tea. Fantastic for coating and soothing sore, scratchy throats, honey is also loaded with antioxidants and phytonutrients that make it a potent antimicrobial ingredient used to help ward off bacteria, viruses, and funguses. Using honey to help promote wellness is called apitherapy. Honey is also used to treat seasonal allergies. If you take a teaspoon of local honey daily, when allergy season comes around you will not be hit as hard with red, watery eyes and sneezing, as your body will have developed a greater resistance to the pollen. Say bye-bye to Claritin.

VANILLA CAMU CAMU CAKE

Makes 12 Servings

Camu camu can do wonders for your vitamin C levels, energy, and skin. Below, you get to maximize the magic in a classic dessert that you can serve the whole family—kids, grannies, postmen, babysitters, and dog walkers included. Everyone deserves a pick-me-up.

Ingredients:

1 cup Truvia Baking Blend

½ cup butter

2 eggs

1 teaspoon vanilla extract

1 teaspoon camu camu extract

1½ cups all-purpose flour

1¾ teaspoons baking powder

½ cup milk

Preparation:

1 Preheat oven to 350°F. Grease and flour a 9 x 9-inch pan or line a muffin pan with paper liners.

2 In a medium bowl, cream together the Truvia Baking Blend and butter. Beat in the eggs, one at a time, then stir in the vanilla, followed by the camu camu extract. Combine the flour and baking powder, add them to the creamed mixture, and mix well. Finally, stir in the milk until the batter is smooth. Pour or spoon the batter into the prepared pan or muffin tins.

3 For cake, bake for 30 to 40 minutes in the preheated oven. For cupcakes, bake 20 to 25 minutes. Cake is done when it springs back to the touch.

BORBA FRIGID

Makes 4 Servings

---

*T*his is one of my favorite light desserts that I invented in my home kitchen. I find that if I gather up ingredients that are in the same taste-bud family, throw in some superfoods and my go-to mix of Truvia Baking Blend, I can produce a new and improved version of something that I'd been eating for years prior that did nothing extra for my skin. Always be open to experimentation, follow your instinct or your favorite nutrition guides, and you may just be pleasantly surprised by what you can dream up.

Ingredients:

8 cups chopped, seeded watermelon—low-calorie superfruit
1½ teaspoons lime juice
1 cup light honey
½ teaspoon ground cardamom—source of iron and manganese
½ package unflavored gelatin
½ cup nonfat plain yogurt
12 mint leaves

Preparation:

1 Place the watermelon and lime juice in a blender and purée.

2 Set a colander over a large bowl and pour the puréed watermelon through, separating the juice from the pulp.

3 Place the juice, honey, cardamom, and gelatin in a large saucepan over medium to high heat for 3 to 4 minutes. Remove from the heat and let cool until it solidifies. Pour into a shallow pan or ice cube tray and freeze to the slush point (about 1¼ hours).

4 Whisk the yogurt into the watermelon slush and then return it to the freezer. Freeze until solid (about 2 hours). Stir every hour to break up the ice crystals.

5 To serve, cut the sherbet into large chunks and purée very briefly in a blender or food processor. Spoon into dessert glasses, garnish with mint leaves, and serve.

ALMOND-OAT SHORTCAKES
with STRAWBERRIES

Makes 6 Shortcakes

*H*ere you get extra nutritional value by mixing oats and almonds into the biscuit dough. Oats provide nutrients, fiber, and beneficial phytochemicals, ensuring a wide range of health benefits, including lower cholesterol. These baby cakes have lots of texture and the almonds are high in monounsaturated fats—the same type of health-promoting fats in olive oil, which have been associated with a reduced risk of heart disease. There are quite a few steps to follow in the preparation of this gorgeous dessert, but the result is well worth it, and you're a fabulous baker anyway, so it's no sweat!

Ingredients:

1 cup all-purpose flour

½ cup old-fashioned oats

⅓ cup slivered almonds—high nutrition

⅓ cup plus 1 tablespoon Truvia Baking Blend, divided

2 teaspoons baking powder

½ teaspoon kosher salt

6 tablespoons (¾ stick) chilled unsalted butter, cut into ½-inch cubes

1 cup chilled heavy cream, divided, plus more for brushing—lactic acid

1½ teaspoons vanilla extract, divided

4 cups hulled, sliced fresh strawberries—low-cal superfruit

1 tablespoon Grand Marnier or other orange liqueur, optional

Preparation:

1 Preheat the oven to 375°F. Line a baking sheet with parchment paper.

2 Pulse the flour, oats, almonds, ⅓ cup of Truvia Baking Blend, baking powder, and salt in a food processor until finely ground.

3 Add the butter; pulse until only pea-size pieces remain. Add ½ cup of cream and 1 teaspoon of vanilla; pulse until large moist clumps form. Transfer to a work surface.

4 Knead until the dough comes together. Pat into a 4 x 6-inch rectangle. Halve lengthwise, then crosswise into thirds. Arrange on the prepared baking sheet. Brush with cream; sprinkle with ½ tablespoon Truvia Baking Blend.

5 Bake, rotating the sheet halfway through cooking, until golden brown around the edges and a tester inserted into the center comes out clean, about 20 minutes.

6 Set the biscuits on a wire rack, let cool. Note: Biscuits can be made 8 hours ahead, cooled, and stored in an airtight container at room temperature.

7 Combine the strawberries and the Grand Marnier, if using, in a large bowl. Toss to coat. Let the strawberries sit, tossing often, until the juices release.

8 Whisk ½ cup of cream, ½ tablespoon of Truvia Baking Blend, and ½ teaspoon of vanilla in a small bowl until peaks form.

9 Cut warm or room-temp biscuits in half; place the bottom halves on plates. Place whipped cream and strawberries over the bottom halves. Top with the remaining biscuit halves.

APPLESAUCE CAKE

Makes 12 Servings
---

*T*his is a quick and easy dessert you will be proud to serve or give, or even eat for breakfast thanks to its health-promoting ingredients such as soy, tofu, raisins, and spices like clove, nutmeg, and cinnamon.

Ingredients:

1¾ cups Truvia Baking Blend
1½ cups all-purpose flour
1 cup sifted soy flour
1½ teaspoons baking soda
¼ teaspoon baking powder
1 teaspoon salt
1 teaspoon cinnamon—anti-inflammatory
½ teaspoon cloves—antiseptic properties
½ teaspoon allspice—digestive stimulant
½ teaspoon nutmeg—antimicrobial properties
½ cup soft silken tofu—reduces cholesterol
2 cups applesauce, chunky style
½ cup vegetable oil
1 cup chopped raisins

Preparation:

1 Preheat the oven to 350°F. In a large bowl, mix thoroughly the Truvia Baking Blend, all-purpose flour, soy flour, baking soda, baking powder, salt, and spices.

2 In a separate bowl, beat the tofu until creamy; add the applesauce and vegetable oil; mix well. Add the tofu mixture to the dry ingredients and beat until well blended. Fold in the raisins.

3 Pour the batter into a greased and floured 9 x 13-inch cake pan. Bake for 45 to 50 minutes.

GOJI BERRY-WALNUT MUFFIN CRUNCH

Makes 12 to 16 Muffins

G oji berries have long been regarded as one of the most nutrient-rich superfoods on the planet! They have an outstanding amount of poly-saccharides to help build the immune system, as well as a full range of antioxidants that provide greater health, vitality, longevity, energy, and stamina—and they are phenomenal for the skin. I even have a bag of dark chocolate covered goji berries in my car for when I'm stuck in traffic! Eating foods high in antioxidants may slow the aging process by minimizing damage from free radicals that injure cells and damage DNA. Rich in vitamin A, and a good source of vitamin C, these berries additionally possess over 20 trace minerals and vitamins including zinc, iron, phosphorus, riboflavin (B_2), vitamin E, and carotenoids, which include beta-carotene. And to put things in perspective on just how powerful the little goji berry is, ounce per ounce it contains more vitamin C than oranges, more beta-carotene than carrots, and more iron than soybeans or spinach. Goji berries are a truly remarkable food, the gold standard for glowing skin and inside-out beauty. Go gojis!

Ingredients:

¼ cup toasted and coarsely chopped walnuts
3 small carrots, finely peeled
1 small apple, peeled and grated
1⅓ cups buckwheat flour
½ cup Truvia Baking Blend
½ teaspoon baking soda
1 teaspoon baking powder
¼ teaspoon salt
1 teaspoon ground cinnamon
¾ cup goji berry raisins—superfood
½ cup coconut, optional
2 large eggs
½ cup canola oil—lowest saturated fat content of any oil commonly consumed
½ teaspoon pure vanilla extract—can help with skin challenges or
   topical wounds

Preparation:

1 Preheat the oven to 350°F.

2 Line twelve to sixteen muffin cups.

3 Toast the walnuts on a baking sheet for about 8 minutes or until lightly browned. Let cool and then chop coarsely.

4 Peel and finely grate the carrots and apple. Set aside.

5 In a large bowl, whisk together the flour, Truvia Baking Blend, baking soda, baking powder, salt, and ground cinnamon.

6 Stir in the toasted walnuts, goji berries, and coconut, if using.

7 In a separate bowl whisk together the eggs, oil, and vanilla extract. Fold the wet ingredients, along with the grated carrot and apple, into the flour mixture, stirring just until moistened.

8 Evenly divide the batter between the prepared muffin cups and bake on the center rack for 20 to 25 minutes or until a toothpick inserted in the center comes out clean.

9 Remove from the oven and let cool on a wire rack. Remove the muffins from the pan after about 10 minutes and cool.

SWEET GOJI YOGURT MEDLEY

Makes 4 Servings

S *ome of the elements in this mix may be new to you. At some point in our lives, everything is new once, right? Now is a great time to get familiar with these nutrient-rich ingredients that contribute to improved health and a unique low-calorie beauty-enhancing dessert you can offer friends and family to show them you care. With no added sugar, this is an unconventional dessert, or breakfast, that is unprocessed and pure. Crunch down on goji berries and know you are doing your body a world of good.*

Ingredients:

⅓ cup chopped almonds

⅓ cup soaked and sprouted sunflower seeds

⅓ cup goji berries—low-cal superfruit

½ cup chopped dried apricots

½ cup chopped dried apples

⅓ cup chopped dried black mission figs—fiber; surprising sweetness serves
    as a sugar substitute

½ cup shredded coconut

1 teaspoon cinnamon

½ teaspoon cloves

¼ teaspoon fresh nutmeg

1 teaspoon orange zest

Pinch Himalayan crystal salt

2½ cups Greek yogurt—probiotic/good intestinal bacteria

⅓ cup blueberries, as garnish—low-cal superfruit

Preparation:

   Coarsely grind the almonds and sunflower seeds in a food processor with the S-blade and set aside. Blend all the other ingredients, except for the yogurt and blueberries, until the fruit is chunky. Stir the nut mixture into the Greek yogurt, add in the chunky fruit mixture, and serve with whole blueberries on top.

SWEET COUSCOUS with ALMOND MILK

*T*his mellow dessert is known in Africa as seffa. Almond milk can be used in cakes, breads, muffins, and other baked goods to replace dairy. It's an easy swap because with almond milk, there is no need to adjust the quantity. The substitution can affect the baking time, however, so you may need to remove your dish from the oven a few minutes earlier than the recipe indicates.

Ingredients:

1 cup almond milk

½ cup very finely chopped or ground blanched almonds

4 tablespoons butter

1½ cups couscous—selenium

Salt

¼ cup raisins

¼ cup chopped dried apricot—fiber

¼ cup chopped dates

¼ cup Truvia Baking Blend, to taste

½ teaspoon ground cinnamon, to taste

Preparation:

1 Combine the milk and almonds in a saucepan with a lid and bring to a boil over medium-high heat.

2 Turn off the heat, cover, and let it sit while you proceed with the recipe.

3 Put 2 tablespoons of the butter in a medium saucepan and turn the heat to medium-low.

4 When the butter melts, add the couscous and cook, stirring, for 1 minute.

5 Add 2¼ cups water and a pinch of salt to the couscous.

6 Bring to a boil, then turn the heat down very low.

7 Cover and cook until all the liquid is absorbed, about 7 to 12 minutes.

8 While the couscous is cooking, soak the raisins, apricots, and dates in warm water for about 20 minutes to rehydrate them. Drain.

9 Pour the couscous into a large serving bowl and stir in the remaining butter along with the drained fruit.

10 Fluff the couscous and break up any lumps.

11 Add the Truvia Baking Blend and cinnamon, and stir; taste and adjust seasonings, if needed.

12 Strain the almond milk and pour over the couscous and serve.

SOY-BERRY COBBLER

Makes 4 to 6 Servings

Here you get a classic cobbler with a berry good-for-you twist. Antioxidants in body-strengthening soymilk and soy flour provide energy to keep your body functioning at its finest. Soy is naturally high in essential fatty acids, proteins, fiber, vitamins, and minerals, and this powerful triumvirate of free-radical fighting berries is sure to satisfy a tangy tart-sweet craving.

Ingredients: Fruit Filling

2 cup blackberries—low-cal superfruit

2 cups blueberries—low-cal superfruit

2 cups raspberries—low-cal superfruit

½ cup raw sugar

¼ cup soy flour blend*

Crust

1½ cups soy flour blend

3 tablespoons Truvia Baking Blend, plus 1 teaspoon for topping

3 teaspoons baking powder

¼ teaspoon salt

6 tablespoons margarine

⅔ cup soy milk

1 egg, beaten

*To make soy flour blend: Combine and mix 7 cups of all-purpose flour and 1 cup of soy flour. Use as needed for the above recipe and keep the rest in a canister for use in any recipe that calls for all-purpose flour as an ingredient.

Preparation: Fruit Filling

1 Place the blackberries, blueberries, and raspberries in a large mixing bowl.

2 Combine the raw sugar and soy flour blend in a small bowl, then add to the fruit mixture, lightly coating the fruit. Place the coated fruit in a greased 8 x 8-inch square baking dish.

Crust

3 In a large bowl, combine the soy flour blend, Truvia Baking Blend, baking powder, and salt. Cut in the margarine until blended. Add the soy milk and blend until the mixture forms a soft dough.

4 Place the dough between 2 pieces of parchment paper and roll out to fit the top of the fruit in the baking dish. Place the dough on top of the fruit, brush with the beaten egg, and sprinkle with 1 teaspoon of Truvia Baking Blend. Bake at 350°F for 35 to 40 minutes or until golden brown.

PUMPKIN CHEESECAKE WEDGES

A creamy, luscious snack is a decadent way to incorporate high-nutrient pumpkin into your dessert repertoire outside of Halloween or Thanksgiving time. Pumpkin is great year-round, and it's loaded with protein, vitamin A for skin clarity, antioxidants, and omega-3 fatty acids for smoother looking skin. If you have sweet potatoes on hand, you can use them instead of pumpkin; they will take on the sweetness of the other ingredients.

Ingredients: Crust

1 cup animal-cracker crumbs—you can use gluten-free
    cracker crumbs

1 teaspoon flaxseed meal—alpha-linolenic acid can help reduce LDL,
    the bad cholesterol

4 tablespoons liquid coconut oil or melted butter

Filling

1 (8-ounce) package of Neufchatel cheese or cream cheese,
    at room temperature

1½ cups pumpkin purée—rich in antioxidants

2 teaspoons vanilla

1 cup Truvia Baking Blend

2 eggs

1 teaspoon cinnamon

¼ teaspoon salt

Preparation: Crust

1 Preheat the oven to 350°F.

2 Make the crust by blending the animal-cracker crumbs, flaxseed
    meal, and oil until thoroughly combined.

3 Press the mixture into a 9-inch pie pan and bake for 5 minutes.
    Let cool.

Filling

1 Start the filling by combining all the ingredients in a high-speed blender (such as a Vitamix) or food processor and blending until smooth and creamy.

2 Pour the filling into the prepared crust.

3 Bake for 45 to 55 minutes, or until the middle is barely set. Allow to cool before slicing.

The Mighty Vitamix

This is not an inexpensive appliance, but I have had mine for ten years, and counting, and it serves me well for many different kinds of foods and recipes. It is an investment, to be sure, but a high-quality one that will go the distance for you down the line. It takes the place of a blender *and* food processor, all in one. So, in addition to cancelling out two space-taking appliances, it also does double duty. Worth your consideration!

PINEAPPLE CAKE with
CREAM CHEESE–GINGER FROSTING

Makes 12 Servings

A fun and easy dessert to make with kids that's finger-licking good with a few sneaked-in ingredients that are good for kids, too. Goes down nicely with a hot mug of soothing green tea, which contains L-theanine, a known calming compound, for focused, even-keeled energy (without the peaks and valleys of caffeine from coffee and espresso).

Ingredients: Cake

2 eggs

1 (20-ounce) can crushed pineapple in juice—superfruit that softens skin and fights free radicals; it also makes a powerful raw food face mask

2 cups flour

1 cup Truvia Baking Blend

1 cup brown sugar

2 teaspoons baking soda

1 cup chopped walnuts—protein

Frosting

1 (3-ounce) package cream cheese

¼ cup butter

1 teaspoon vanilla

½ teaspoon camu camu extract or powder—off-the-charts vitamin C

2 cups powdered sugar

½ teaspoon powdered ginger

Preparation:

Preheat the oven to 350°F. Combine all the cake ingredients and pour into an ungreased, 13 x 9-inch Pyrex pan and bake for 45 to 50 minutes. Combine the frosting ingredients and spread on the pineapple cake once it has cooled.

SPEEDY SCRUMPTIOUS SORBET

Makes 4 Servings

This light, refreshing, frozen dessert is always a great option when you want something sweet without calories from fat. Getting in your superfruit antioxidants is a breeze when you're spooning away at a cold dish of sorbet.

Ingredients:

2 cups strawberries
2 cups blueberries
½ cup Truvia Baking Blend
2 tablespoons powdered sugar
Pinch of salt

Preparation:

Blend strawberries and blueberries with ½ cup of water. Add Truvia Baking Blend, powdered sugar, and a pinch of salt. Purée until smooth. Pour the puréed berry mixture through a sieve to strain seeds and skin, and then put the mixture in a freezer-safe container. Freeze for around 2 hours. Allow it to thaw a few minutes before serving.

NO-BAKE BROWNIE TRUFFLES

Makes 15 Truffles

These luscious sweet truffles are perfect after a long hard day. They're an easy way to get hefty doses of protein, minerals, vitamins, and anti-oxidants, and a touch of comfort, too. Make them on the weekend so they are ready to eat during the week. These are fun for small children to scoop, shape, decorate, and, of course, devour.

Ingredients:

1 cup almonds (no salt added)

15 dried pitted dates (vitamins A, B_6, C, E, K)

⅔ cup unsweetened cocoa powder, plus extra for dusting

1 tablespoon honey—antiseptic properties

2 tablespoons water

2 tablespoons cocoa, or confectioner's sugar, or finely chopped dried fruit, or finely chopped nuts, or unsweetened flaked coconut for rolling, optional

Preparation:

1 Add the almonds to a high-speed blender (such as a Vitamix) or a food processor. Pulse until ground.

2 Add the dates, cocoa powder, honey, and water to the almond mixture. Pulse until the mixture just begins to form a sticky mass. (You may need to add a few drops of additional water to get the right consistency.)

3 Using clean hands or cookie scoops, make balls the size of golf balls.

4 If you'd like to add a coating, put cocoa, confectioner's sugar, finely chopped dried fruit or nuts, and/or flaked coconut on a plate. Drop the balls onto the plate and roll to coat.

CHOCOLATE CANDY CRUNCHIES

Makes 12 Servings

W*hile these look and taste like candy, there is no added refined sugar. All the sweetness comes from the raisins and chocolate, two powerful antioxidants. Since you are now an expert in the fact that everything that goes into our bodies should nourish us, you can relax and enjoy these "crunchies" because they certainly do the trick. When I put these out at parties, or offer them on the dessert table, there are never any leftovers. Perfect for any festive occasion.*

Ingredients:

½ cup toasted walnuts

½ cup soft raisins

½ teaspoon ground flaxseeds

½ cup organic cornflakes—gluten-free

1 cup semisweet chocolate chips

Preparation:

1 Chop the nuts finely.

2 Toss the nuts into a bowl with the raisins, flaxseed, and cornflakes.

3 Gently melt the chocolate chips in the top of a double boiler.

4 Pour the chocolate into the bowl with the nut mixture, and stir all the ingredients together.

5 Drop the mixture onto parchment paper by using a small tablespoon.

6 Chill in the refrigerator for 1 hour.

OLIVE OIL ICE CREAM

Makes 1 Quart

*I*ce cream is a delightful indulgence, but olive oil ice cream is a treat you can feel good about eating. Ingredients that are good for your skin make up for those extra calories, which you'll burn off at the gym anyway, right? In a basic custard base, olive oil substitutes for some of the heavy cream, as you will see below. The key to achieving a yummy ice cream is great-tasting olive oil, and it is also a major skin-care ingredient. You don't want to use a peppery, grassy, or herbal olive oil; go with a fruity-flavored, sweeter-aroma type. This innovative take on America's favorite dessert has actually been in the gourmet food world for ten years.

Ingredients:

1⅓ cups whole milk—vitamin D

½ cup Truvia Baking Blend

Pinch salt

6 large egg yolks

1½ cups heavy cream—lactic acid

1 sticky vanilla bean, scraped inside—contains natural pain relievers to soothe the system

⅔ cup fruity Chilean extra-virgin olive oil—fine and flavorful!

Caramel sauce, as topping

Preparation:

1 Warm the milk, Truvia Baking Blend, and salt in a medium-size saucepan.

2 In a separate medium bowl, whisk the egg yolks. Slowly pour the warm milk mixture into the egg yolks, whisking constantly. Then scrape the warm milk mixture back into the saucepan.

3 Stir the mixture constantly over medium heat with a heatproof spatula, scraping the bottom as you stir, until the mixture thickens to a custardlike consistency and coats the spatula. Turn off the heat when the custard just slightly thickens.

4 Pour the heavy cream and vanilla scrapings into a large bowl and set a mesh strainer on top. Pour the custard through the strainer and stir it into the cream.

5 Whisk the Chilean fruity olive oil into the custard mixture until it's well blended; then stir until cool over an ice bath.

6 Chill the mixture thoroughly in the refrigerator, then freeze it in your ice cream maker according to the manufacturer's instructions. If you don't have an ice cream maker, you can place the mixture in a large Ziploc bag, place rock salt in another bag, and set the mixture right on top of the rock salt. Freeze the mixture thoroughly in the freezer. Top with caramel sauce when ready to eat.

The Power of Pink!

Why is Himalayan salt pink, and what does it do for food? Said to be the purest salt found on earth, these antimicrobial, hand-mined, pink, iodized crystals offer many healing benefits including lowering blood pressure, improving circulation, and detoxing the body of heavy metals. The salt's many hues of pink, red, and white are an indication of its rich and varying mineral and iron content. Standard commercial table salt or cooking salt is often chemically cleaned.

OLIVE OIL and PISTACHIO ICE CREAM

Makes 4 Servings

*A*n oily, sticky true vanilla pod (not a dried-out one from a jar) contributes directly to the hydrating and healing of your skin when incorporated with other skin-nourishing ingredients. Used in this recipe, vanilla works well for your skin alongside the olive oil. This recipe is so simple.

Ingredients:

1 vanilla pod, extracted

5 scoops pistachio ice cream

5 tablespoons extra-virgin olive oil

½ teaspoon sea salt flakes

Preparation:

1 Extract the essence of the vanilla pod by cutting it open, or splitting it lengthwise, and scraping out the vanilla beans.

2 Place the ice cream in a frozen cold bowl with the extracted vanilla.

3 Drizzle with the olive oil and sea salt flakes. Mix and refreeze.

DARK CHOCOLATE WALNUT COOKIE BITES

Makes 36 Cookies
---

*J*oy to the baker who churns out these babies. Soft, brownielike cookies are *sooo satisfying. When it comes to mix-ins, I go for the toasted walnuts, but you can try dried cherries or apricots, pecans, golden raisins, goji berries, white chocolate, or Valrhona. You can dream big with these little cookies.*

Ingredients:

8-ounce dark chocolate baking bar, broken into pieces

2 large eggs—contain high-quality protein and all 9 essential amino acids

¼ teaspoon salt

¼ cup packed brown sugar

¼ cup protein powder (available in any nutrition store)

1 teaspoon vanilla extract

1 cup chopped walnuts, toasted, plus more as garnish

¼ cup all-purpose flour

Preparation:

1 Preheat the oven to 325°F. Grease two baking sheets.

2 Microwave the broken baking bars in a medium, uncovered, microwave-safe bowl on high for 1 minute; stir. If pieces retain some of their original shape, microwave at an additional 10- to 15-second interval, stirring just until melted.

3 Beat the eggs and salt in a small mixer bowl on high speed for 3 minutes or until thick. Add the brown sugar and protein powder; beat for an additional 5 minutes. Beat in the melted chocolate and vanilla extract. Stir in the chopped walnuts and flour.

4 Drop by rounded teaspoonfuls onto the prepared baking sheets. Top the cookies with walnuts.

5 Bake for 8 to 10 minutes or until shiny and set. Cool on baking sheets for 2 minutes; remove to wire racks to cool completely.

STUFFED LYCHEES

*T*his entire creation takes but 15 minutes to prepare. The macadamias and lychees make for an exotic flavor that's rich, creamy, and crunchy— and something interesting to offer as a passed dessert at your unique soiree. For a dinner party, they look beautiful in any of your special-yet-oft-neglected fine glassware dessert bowls or cut-crystal candy dishes.

Ingredients:

2 (20-ounce) cans lychees, pits removed—low-cal superfruit

1 (8-ounce) package cream cheese

1 tablespoon sherry wine

1 dash salt

3 tablespoons chopped macadamia nuts—cholesterol-free

2 tablespoons chopped crystallized ginger
  (shelf stable for up to 2 years)

Preparation:

1 Drain the lychees.

2 For stuffing: In a small bowl of an electric mixer, beat the cream cheese with the sherry and salt until the mixture is creamy. Stir in the remaining ingredients.

3 Stuff the lychees.

EASY AFFOGATO

Makes 1 Serving

*T*his decadent Italian dessert always strikes me as so impressive when I order it at a restaurant, but, in actuality, it is simple to create. The one I make for dinner parties uses frozen yogurt instead of ice cream, which goes over well with guests who may be "watching their line."

Ingredients:

½ cup vanilla frozen yogurt

½ tablespoon Kahlua coffee liqueur

2 tablespoons hot espresso

Preparation:

Scoop frozen yogurt into a serving dish. Stir the liqueur into the espresso, then pour over the frozen yogurt. Serve immediately.

 ## Dimpled-Skin Caffeine Scrub

Caffeine is probably the most common ingredient you will find in lotions that fight dimpled skin. Caffeine is a stimulant and vasodilator, which means it opens up blood vessels and helps to reduce fat cells. Although it is a stimulant drug, and therefore one to be taken in moderation, caffeine can help with the breakdown of fat molecules stored in fat cells.

For the scrub:

In a bowl, mix ½ cup of warm coffee grounds with 2 tablespoons of olive oil. Take to the bathroom (stand in the tub) and, using pressure, briskly loofah the mixture in circles on problem skin areas that need increased circulation. Next, wrap the area(s) in plastic wrap. Then, using a rolling pin or a bumpy brush, "roll out" the skin by massaging the targeted area briskly. Do this for at least 10 minutes, remove the plastic wrap, and wash off the scrub with warm water. Over time and with consistency, this treatment can be an effective way to smooth out the lumpy appearance of cottage cheese–like skin.

DARK CHOCOLATE and PISTACHIO COOKIES

Makes 2 Dozen Cookies

*P*istachios are the health nut's nut. Why? They're full of vitamin B_6 and copper, which help increase energy. They are high in protein, fiber, and healthy monounsaturated fat, all of which contribute to the slowing of the body's carbohydrate absorption. Eating up to 3 ounces of pistachios a day can help raise your level of good cholesterol (HDL). And they're fun to crack open, too.

Ingredients:

1 stick unsalted butter, room temperature
½ cup Truvia Baking Blend
½ cup packed brown sugar
1 large egg
1 teaspoon vanilla extract

1¼ cups all-purpose flour
½ teaspoon baking soda
¼ teaspoon salt
1½ cups dark chocolate chips
1 cup coarsely chopped pistachios

Preparation:

1 Place a rack in the upper third of the oven and preheat the oven to 300°F.

2 Line two baking sheets with parchment paper and set aside.

3 In the bowl of an electric stand mixer fitted with a paddle attachment, beat the butter, Truvia Baking Blend, and brown sugar together until pale, about 4 minutes. Add the egg and beat for about 1 minute. Add the vanilla extract and beat to incorporate.

4 In a medium bowl, whisk together the flour, baking soda, and salt. Add the flour mixture all at once to the butter mixture. Beat on low speed until just incorporated. Finally, mix in the chocolate chips and nuts.

5 Scoop the cookie dough by 2 tablespoonfuls onto baking sheets, about 2 inches apart.

6 Bake for 18 minutes, or until just golden brown. Remove from the oven and allow to cool before removing to a wire rack to cool completely.

KEY LIME PIE with AVOCADO and COCONUT FILLING

Makes 10 Servings

Hero Recipe!

An innovative recipe that is across-the-board good for you. Hard to believe it's a dessert. Your friends and family will likely say the same!

Ingredients: Crust

6 pitted dates—calcium, fiber, amino acids, sulfur

1 cup macadamia nuts

1 cup walnuts

½ teaspoon vanilla

Pinch of salt

Filling

¾ cup lime juice—vitamin C

½ cup honey

1 cup mashed avocado —low-cal superfruit

¼ cup coconut milk

2 teaspoons vanilla

Pinch of salt

½ cup coconut oil

Whipped Cream

2 cups whipping cream

½ teaspoon vanilla

1 teaspoon Truvia Baking Blend

Garnish

Lime slices

Raspberries—low-cal superfruit

Mint leaves

Coconut shreds

Preparation: Crust

1 Process the dates in a food processor until they become a paste. Then add the nuts and remaining ingredients and process until crumbly.

2 Place the mixture in a 12-inch springform pan and work it up the sides to create a thick crust.

Filling

Blend the filling ingredients in a blender until smooth. Pour into the piecrust you made in Step 2. Freeze for 1 hour.

Whipped Cream

While the pie freezes, whip the cream until it forms soft peaks. Remove the pie, spread the whipped cream on top, and then put the pie back in the freezer for at least 2 hours more.

Assemble and Garnish

When you are ready to serve, remove the pie from the freezer and let it sit for 1 hour to soften before serving. Garnish with lime slices, raspberries, mint leaves, and shredded coconut.

LEMON CREAM PIE

Makes 8 Servings

When life gives you lemons, you make . . . cream pie! Lemons are a citrus wonder that aid the body in flushing out toxins as well as jump-starting the digestive tract with enzymatic processes. Lemons also aid the liver in its cleansing processes. Lemons contain citric acid, calcium, magnesium, vitamin C, bioflavonoids, pectin, and limonene that promote immunity and fight infection. To jump-start any day, start out your morning with a warm glass of lemon water; it's a good cleansing detox drink for your body, and a great ritual for morning time. In this recipe you get some lemon love and a gelatin fix, too.

Ingredients:

¼ cup water

1 (4-ounce) package of sugar-free lemon gelatin—low-cal

2 (6-ounce) Yoplait Light fat-free lemon yogurts, or the brand you prefer

8 ounces of heavy cream

1 (9-inch) graham cracker crust

Preparation:

1 Boil the water and pour into a large mixing bowl.

2 Pour in the gelatin and whisk until dissolved.

3 Add the yogurt and whisk together with the gelatin, mix thoroughly.

4 Beat in the heavy cream and transfer the mix to the graham cracker crust.

5 Refrigerate for 4 hours.

 Simple Lemon Facial for Exfoliation

After washing your face with warm water, pat it dry with a fresh towel. Next, squeeze the juice from a lemon into a bowl. (It doesn't matter if the seeds fall in.) Soak a cotton ball or cotton square in the lemon juice. Hold the moistened cotton ball between your fingers while drizzling some sugar over its surface. After the sugar soaks in for a minute and "crystallizes," use the cotton ball to gently exfoliate the entire face, using a circular motion. This exfoliating scrub contains alpha hydroxy and beta hydroxy acids, which remove upper dead skin layers on your face, leaving skin feeling smooth.

CARAMELIZED APPLES

Makes 6 Servings

The classic treat of every childhood beach boardwalk and circus experience gets a makeover. These apples are served in a bowl rather than eaten off a stick. I've left out the sticky hard caramel coating that's tough on teeth; these are cooked to the point that their natural fruit juices caramelize. You also get more of a "pie-flavor" effect because this recipe calls for three different types of apples that all bring something unique to the plate. Lemon is clarifying and cinnamon brings blood and nutrients to the skin surface to assist with eye-area puffiness and a host of other beauty challenges.

Ingredients:

3 tablespoons butter

5 spicy-sweet, crisp apples (Jonagold, Crispin, Honeycrisp), peeled and cut into ½-inch cubes

1 tablespoon plus 2 tablespoons Truvia Baking Blend, divided

½ teaspoon ground cinnamon—antibacterial

¼ teaspoon lemon zest

⅓ cup apple cider—a health tonic good for dry skin

½ teaspoon cornstarch, optional

Preparation:

1 Melt the butter in a large skillet over medium heat. Add the apples to the pan and sprinkle with 1 tablespoon of Truvia Baking Blend. Sauté the apples, stirring frequently, for 6 to 8 minutes, until they just start to turn tender.

2 Sprinkle the apples with the remaining Truvia Baking Blend, cinnamon, and lemon zest. Toss the mixture gently and cook over medium heat for an additional 2 minutes, until the sugar begins to caramelize and the apples are crisp yet tender.

3 Transfer the apples from the skillet to a serving bowl with a slotted spoon. Turn the heat to high and add the apple cider to the skillet, scraping up any browned apple bits. Reduce the heat slightly and allow the cider and the pan juices to simmer for 1 to 3 minutes, until the sauce has reduced and thickened slightly. If you desire a thicker sauce, dissolve the cornstarch in a teaspoon of water, stir it into the sauce, and allow it to thicken for a moment. Pour the finished sauce over the warm apples and serve immediately.

VANILLA-PUMPKIN PUDDING

Makes 2 Servings

*I*f you like the flavor of vanilla extract, and I do so much that I even put a few drops in my drip coffee, this vanilla-pumpkin pudding makes for a yummy breakfast or snack that tastes just like pumpkin pie filling. It's an easy treat to make that will satisfy, give you energy, and power you through your morning. The key ingredient is canned pumpkin, which is low in calories, high in fiber, and bursting with beta-carotene. Some people only eat pumpkin during wintertime holidays; I like it year-round and recommend you add canned pumpkin to your kitchen pantry.

Ingredients:

6 ounces nonfat yogurt, vanilla flavor

⅓ cup canned 100 percent pure pumpkin purée (no added sugar)

1 dash ground cinnamon

1 tablespoon chopped, toasted nuts (almonds, walnuts, or pecans, optional)
   —protein

Preparation:

In a small bowl, blend together the yogurt, pumpkin, and cinnamon until creamy. Top with nuts, if desired.

MINI CHOCO CHEW-CHEW CAKES

Makes 24 Minicakes

*F*ight fat while you snack? In this recipe, creamy thick Greek yogurt offers a combination of protein, fat, and healthy carbs that help burn belly fat—twice as much protein as other yogurts do, so you'll feel more satisfied.

Ingredients:

½ cup reduced-fat cream cheese, room temperature

2 tablespoons Truvia Baking Blend

½ cup nonfat plain Greek yogurt

½ teaspoon vanilla extract

¾ cup unbleached all-purpose flour

¼ cup unsweetened cocoa powder, plus more for dusting—antioxidants

½ teaspoon baking soda

½ cup granulated sugar

3 tablespoons unsalted butter

1 egg white

½ cup skim milk, divided

Preparation:

1 Beat the cream cheese and Truvia Baking Blend in a bowl with an electric mixer on high until smooth. Add the yogurt and vanilla; beat until well combined.

2 Coat three baking sheets with vegetable oil cooking spray. Heat the oven to 400°F. Whisk the flour, cocoa powder, and baking soda in a second bowl.

3 Beat the sugar and butter with an electric mixer on high in a third bowl until combined; add the egg white and beat until the mixture is thick and pale yellow.

4 Add half the flour mixture to the sugar mixture; beat until just combined. Add ¼ cup of milk; beat on low speed until combined. Repeat with the remaining flour mixture and remaining ¼ cup of milk.

5 Transfer the batter into a large resealable bag; squeeze the batter into a corner of the bag and clip the small corner to make a piping bag. Squeeze sixteen lines of batter, 4 inches long and 1 inch apart, onto each baking sheet. Bake until the centers spring back to the touch, 5 to 7 minutes. Cool on a wire rack.

6 Spread half the cakes with cream cheese filling; top with a second cake to make sandwiches and dust with cocoa powder, if desired. Serve immediately, or store in the refrigerator for up to 3 days.

 ## "Mocha" Hydrating Body Scrub

Superhydration and moisture retention are essential for smooth, supple skin that is soft to the touch. Cocoa powder and coffee grounds improve circulation, especially when rubbed over legs and thighs as an exfoliant. If only all those mocha lattes I drink had the same effect! You can use the coffee grounds from your morning brew, but I think fresh unsoaked grounds are even more effective as they retain the caffeine, which in this treatment is needed for circulation. Almond oil is high in vitamin E, which helps your skin retain its moisture, and it is a powerful antioxidant. Shea butter is extremely hydrating, has anti-inflammatory properties, and you can buy it inexpensively at your local 99-cent store. For this home-spa treatment, you'll need:

3 tablespoons almond oil
1 teaspoon coffee grounds
1 teaspoon cocoa powder
1 tablespoon shea butter

Using a small bowl, mix all the ingredients together. While in the shower, and pores are clean and open, apply the scrub to targeted areas and rub in a circular motion. Try to stay out of the shower stream while rubbing in this hydrating, natural body scrub. Rinse thoroughly and you will have smooth, supple skin. Maybe you can even say, "Spanx, no thanks. I'm good as I am, and getting better, *baby!*"

Now that you have learned some delicious recipes for desserts, snacks, and other little lovelies, I hope you will experiment with them and pass them along to your friends, too. Remember: knowledge is power, and, if you have knowledge, you should always allow others to light their candles in it.

In addition to eating the foods you love and trying out different hair- and skin-care treatments using that food's ingredients, I hope that by now you are starting to get a feel for what foods and supplements benefit your skin internally and externally. If you can commit some of this information to memory it will empower your next jaunt to the supermarket, restaurant, or health food store. Share what you are learning with your loved ones; it's a great way to reinforce the facts in your brain and hear yourself sticking to the plan of tweaking meals, snacks, and desserts with beauty boosters and hero ingredients. You will find yourself at home with smart foods that power your body, skin, and mind! I firmly believe that we are what we eat. What's inside is projected outward, so keep up the good work and keep going for the gorgeous.

Cocktails and Mocktails

Chapter 7

Now that we've graduated from desserts for your every taste bud's desire, we can hit the hard stuff! That *other indulgence* so many of us take pleasure in from time to time, or more frequently than that—happy hour, the cold frosty one, libation station—however we choose to call it, alcohol is a part of life and it can be a pleasure to unwind and socialize with, bar none. In fact, I long for those festive nights when I can appreciate and savor a fine bottle of wine with a friend, or a spicy jalapeño margarita. The antioxidants and other nutrients infused into my specialized drinks have undeniable health benefits, and getting them via libation is better than not getting them at all. If you are going to partake in a cocktail or glass of wine, why not add skin-friendly ingredients into the mix? My theory is, if you're going to drink spirits you might as well get a beauty boost while you're at it so you can confidently say, "Bottoms Up." One drink is usually considered to measure as a medium glass of wine, a 1.5 ounce shot of spirits, or a can or bottle of beer. All of those have roughly similar amounts of pure alcohol in them. For most folks, one to two drinks will suffice for a good time, so please drink in moderation and never beyond your comfort level. These drinks can offer skin-health benefits with a newfangled twist. You can make your own signature cocktails, too, the ones you tout at your swanky soirees. But remember, no amount of alcohol is going to hydrate your skin—and glowing skin requires hydration—so be sure to drink a minimum of 12 ounces of water after your cocktails and get a good night's sleep, too, if you can!

In this chapter you'll also get my mocktail recipes for when you choose to pass on the alcohol but you still hanker for the taste and ritual of the cocktail experience.

The palate pleasers in this chapter are mostly a digression from the everyday beverage habits I recommend. For all my readers, teetotalers or other, I share with you the two ways I like to consider my beverages: cocktails for Fundays and nonalcoholic mocktails for Sundays (but they still taste indulgent so you can sip, gulp, and thrive).

If you're out on the town or at a party in someone's home, remember to alternate cocktail and water every round to avoid a dull hangover and extra calories. If you want to drink less water (and remain clearheaded), you can drink *mock*tails instead. As their name implies, these bevvies only "mock" the real drinks and are nonalcoholic; the choice of course is yours whether to include booze or not.

TOP 5 Heroes of the Beverage Universe

Strawberries/Pomegranate—antioxidants.

Ginger—excellent for digestion, good source of manganese, fights infection.

Lemons/Limes—tangy sources of vitamin C; detoxifying.

Mint and/or Spearmint—add refreshing flavor, aid relaxation, preventative against colds and flu.

Hot Sauce—the cloudier, the better. Traditional hot sauces are just *infused* with chile seeds. The more dense and cloudy ones are made with crushed seeds for a more potent and beneficial product.

FIZZY POM-POM

Makes 4 Servings

Pomegranate is a free-radical killer and makes for a killer cocktail. Mixed with sparkling wine, it is refreshing and totally delightful.

Ingredients:

8 ounces pomegranate liqueur

6 ounces pomegranate juice

1 bottle sparkling wine

1 pomegranate, seeds for garnish

Preparation:

Combine the pomegranate liqueur and pomegranate juice. Pour the mixture into champagne glasses and top it with sparkling wine. Drop pomegranate seeds into the champagne glasses for garnish.

SPICED RED WINE

M uch to wine about on this Funday! Skin-friendly grapeseed extract and reservatrol are two powerful antioxidants contained in red wine. In moderation, vino tinto has long been thought to increase levels of good cholesterol and protect the heart against artery damage. This recipe for spiced red wine can be enjoyed any time of year, but I tend to make it during the colder months.

Ingredients:

1 bottle red wine (such as cabernet or merlot)

8 tablespoons brown sugar

1 orange peel

1 grapefruit peel

10 cloves

2 cinnamon sticks, plus 4 to garnish

Preparation:

1 Combine the wine and sugar in a large pot over medium-low heat, stirring occasionally until the sugar is dissolved.

2 Add the orange and grapefruit peels, cloves, and 2 cinnamon sticks. Heat the mixture for 20 minutes, but don't allow the wine to boil.

3 Strain the wine through a fine sieve and let it cool. Serve garnished with cinnamon sticks.

CRAN-PECTIN COSMO

Makes 6 to 8 Servings

I n this cosmopolitan take on a popular cocktail, I employ a thickening technique to get the party started, nightclub music optional.

Ingredients:

2 tablespoons (2 envelopes) unflavored pectin gel
  —vegan and more powerful than gelatin

½ cup cold water

1¼ cups cranberry juice

½ cup sugar

¾ cup cold triple sec—vitamin C!

½ cup cold vodka

2 tablespoons lime juice

1 cup fresh raspberries

Preparation:

1 In a large bowl, sprinkle the pectin evenly over the cold water and allow it to absorb the water for 2 minutes.

2 In a saucepan, bring the cranberry juice and sugar just to a boil over medium heat. Remove from the heat, then pour the boiling mixture into the pectin and stir until the gelatin is fully dissolved.

3 Let the mixture cool; stir in the triple sec, vodka, and lime juice.

4 Refrigerate until thickened but not set. Fold in the raspberries. Spoon into six to eight martini glasses. Refrigerate until firm and serve.

SPARKLING GINGER COCKTAILS

I love ginger because it has such a distinct flavor and spicy attitude! It's a powerful root wonder-spice that targets everything from heartburn to migraines and morning sickness. If you are expecting (congratulations!), simply omit the Prosecco from this recipe.

Ingredients:

¾ cup water

½ cup sliced fresh ginger (2 ounces)

¾ cup Truvia Baking Blend, divided

1 tablespoon finely chopped crystallized ginger

2 lemon wedges

2 (750-ml) bottles chilled Prosecco

Preparation:

1 Simmer the water, fresh ginger, and ½ cup of Truvia Baking Blend in a small saucepan, uncovered, for 10 minutes. Remove from the heat and let the ginger syrup steep for 15 minutes.

2 Strain the syrup through a sieve into a bowl, discarding the solids. Chill until cold.

3 Finely grind the crystallized ginger with the remaining ¼ cup Truvia Baking Blend in a blender or food processor, then spread it on a small plate.

4 Run lemon wedges around the rims of glasses, then dip the rims into the Truvia mixture.

5 Put 1 tablespoon of ginger syrup into each glass and top off with Prosecco.

STRAWBERRY MINT SPRITZER

Makes 4 to 6 Servings

T*his sparkling drink is ideal as a refreshing spritzer for a brunch or on a hot summer day; but I also crave it après ski.*

Ingredients:

1 pint strawberries

3 to 4 springs of mint

6 lemons

1 bottle sake (any kind will do)

1 bottle champagne

Ice

Vanilla Truvia

Preparation:

1 Slice the strawberries into vertical slivers, tear the mint leaves roughly, and add both to a large pitcher.

2 Squeeze the juice of 6 lemons and gently muddle (mash/mix together) the ingredients using a wooden spoon. Add equal parts sake and champagne and lots of ice. Squeeze a dropper full of vanilla Truvia into each glass before serving.

Variation: *If you prefer an alcohol-free version, simply substitute sparkling mineral water for the sake and champagne. It's absolutely delicious and will make you feel like a million bucks every time you take a sip! This recipe is great for entertaining—your guests will be raving about it and asking for the ingredients list, guaranteed.*

Strawberry Fields Forever

Strawberries, so bright, juicy, and delicious, are important additions to a warm weather diet. Here's a berry you should eat for the rest of your life! Available in most markets from late April through July, strawberries have off-the-chart levels of vitamin C, plus huge stores of fiber, antioxidants, and other phytonutrients. (They are available out of season but are far less sweet. Use less sweet ones in blended drinks.) Strawberries promote strong eyesight and have powerful anti-inflammatory powers. Eating them fresh out of the package is a no-brainer, but strawberries are also great tossed into smoothies, juices, salads, muffins, quick bread recipes, and even simmered into syrups.

MAJOR BLOODY MARY

Makes 1 Serving

This is the cocktail to get things moving at a lazy Sunday brunch; enhances Saturday night recall!

Ingredients:

1½ ounces lemon vodka

½ cup tomato juice

2 twists juice from lime

3 pinches white pepper

3 pinches celery salt

½ teaspoon Worcestershire sauce

2 to 3 drops Tabasco

Lime slices, for garnish, optional

Preparation:

Pour all the ingredients, adding only *one* twist of lime, into a shaker half full of ice and shake for a minute. Pour into a highball glass fairly full of ice and then add the next twist of lime to the top of the drink. Garnish with a lime slice, if you choose.

BORBA BULLSHOT

Makes 1 Serving

Savory and hearty with a kick, and good for that long brunch with your cousin's family, the Bullshot takes no prisoners.

Ingredients:

2½ ounces vodka

⅛ teaspoon black pepper

5 ounces beef bouillon

1 dash Tabasco

1 dash Worcestershire sauce

1 wedge lemon

Preparation:

Shake all the ingredients except the lemon wedge in a cocktail shaker with ice. Strain into a highball glass full of ice cubes and garnish with the lemon wedge.

MINUS the SINUS

Makes 1 Serving

A stiff shot for knocking out a stuffy head and clearing the nasal passageways. *Note: If you are under the weather, do not drink alcohol in conjunction with cold or flu medications.* In this recipe I use the liquid ratio in "parts." One part means to use a set amount to measure one. It can be a shot glass worth, thimble's worth, ½-cup worth. It depends on how much of the drink you want to make.

Ingredients:

1 part pepper vodka

1 dash Tabasco sauce

1 pinch white pepper

Preparation:

Mix the vodka and Tabasco in a shot glass. Sprinkle the pepper on top.

EL CISNE NEGRO
(THE BLACK SWAN)

Makes 1 Serving

*T*his little devil's got a bite that can sneak up on you so proceed with caution!

Ingredients:

2 ounces tequila
¾ ounce crème de cassis—sweet, red, black-currant flavored liqueur
Ginger ale
1 lime wedge

Preparation:

Stir the tequila and crème de cassis over ice in a chilled Collins glass. Top off with the ginger ale, squeeze the lime wedge over the drink, then drop it into the glass.

THE SPONGE

Makes 1 Serving

*T*ypically, a sponge wrings out, but this one can boost hydration levels to help keep skin smooth and firm. Guava juice contains many nutrients; it is also rich in fiber and lycopene.

Ingredients:

2 ounces vodka
2 ounces guava juice
1 lemon twist, as garnish

Preparation:

In a cocktail shaker filled halfway with ice, combine the vodka and guava juice and shake well. Strain the mixture into a chilled, stemmed cocktail glass and garnish with a lemon twist.

JALAPEÑO-CILANTRO-STRAWBERRY MARGARITA

Makes 1 Serving

I love sweet and savory cocktails. The flavors complement each other in unexpected ways with the appropriate amount of bite and taste-bud tingle. This recipe may awaken the scientist in you; requires advance preparations.

Ingredients:

1 tablespoon organic agave nectar, to rim glass

Sea salt, to rim glass

2 ounces jalapeño-infused silver agave tequila
   (see How to Infuse Beverages sidebar)

2 ounces fresh organic lime juice

3 ounces strawberry mix or purée
   (Maizena makes a good one, so does Nesquik)

1 ounce cilantro water (blend organic cilantro with small amount of fresh water)

1 organic lime, sliced, as garnish

Preparation:

Rim the glass with organic agave nectar and sea salt. Shake together the tequila, lime juice, strawberry mix, and cilantro water in a shaker and strain over fresh ice in a margarita glass. Garnish with a lime wheel.

TIP: Stop the weight! You can gain nearly 5 pounds in one night if you have one-and-a-half sugar-rich cocktails plus a fried appetizer. Imagine how many of us do this late at night when we are out with friends. *Sheesh!*

How to Infuse Beverages

Infusing beverages is a great way to experiment with flavor making. Choose a clean, airtight jar, place the washed ingredients inside the jar (for the Jalapeño-Cilantro-Strawberry Margarita, cut the jalapeño in half), and fill the jar with your beverage of choice. Shake a few times and cover tightly with a lid. Store in a cool, dark place and shake 3 to 5 times a day to activate. After two days, do a taste test. Maybe you want it to set for 3 days; when your infusion has reached a flavor you like, remove the flavoring ingredient(s) from the jar. Use a fine strainer or paper coffee filter to strain the liquid into another clean jar.

MARGARITA HIBISCUS

<u>Makes 2 Servings</u>

An exotic drink with roots that may be from your garden. Hibiscus helps fight cholesterol, and this delicious drink takes a little time to make, but the flavor and effects are worth it. Orange juice yields vitamin C, and agave nectar's low glycemic index does not spike blood sugar the way refined sugars in common cocktails do.

Ingredients:

*For Hibiscus Reduction

2 ounces dried hibiscus leaves/petals

3 ounces water

Truvia Baking Blend, to taste

*For Sour Mix

4 ounces raw agave nectar

4 ounces fresh squeezed orange juice

6 ounces water

*For Margarita Hibiscus

2 ounces Blanco tequila

2 ounces hibiscus reduction*

2 ounces sour mix**

Preparation:

1 To make hibiscus reduction, in a small saucepan over medium heat mix together the hibiscus, water, and Truvia Baking Blend. Simmer for 30 minutes, or until the color has leached from the hibiscus petals. Remove from the heat, and, if the flavor seems too tangy, add a dash more Truvia. Strain the mixture and let it cool.

2 To make the sour mix, stir together the agave nectar, orange juice, and water.

3 To make the cocktail, shake together the tequila, hibiscus reduction, and sour mix. Strain over ice and serve in a wide fancy glass. The end result should be mildly tart and crisp. Sweetness can be adjusted per cocktail by adding more agave nectar. You can also add in a squeeze of fresh lime juice.

SPICY TEQUILA TEA

Makes 1 Serving

*S*urely your granny never sipped tea like this before! The black tea in chai is rich in antioxidants, and cinnamon is thought to decrease fatigue, increase circulation, and sharpen awareness. (Awareness may decrease due to clean-but-mean Ocho Reposado!)

Ingredients:

2 tablespoons agave nectar

1 tablespoon cinnamon

2 ounces Ocho Reposado tequila

2 ounces chai tea

Preparation:

Rim a martini glass with agave nectar and cinnamon. To do this, simply coat the rim of a glass with the agave juice using a fingertip, then "dunk" the rim into any lid filled with the tablespoon of cinnamon. Shake all the remaining ingredients in a cocktail shaker and then strain into the martini glass.

BORBANADE

Makes 1 Serving

I created this when I was in the mood for a refreshing cold lemonade but found myself in the middle of a Funday, so I said, why not pour in some vodka, too?

Ingredients:

1½ ounces vodka

4½ ounces lemonade

1 ounce pomegranate juice

1 teaspoon grenadine

1 lemon, sliced, as garnish

Preparation:

Pour the vodka, lemonade, pomegranate, and grenadine into a tall glass with ice. Stir and garnish with a lemon wheel. Sip, gulp, thrive!

POMEVATION

I f you like rum, this is a delicious mixture replete with vitamin C.

Ingredients:

2 ounces vodka

6 ounces tonic

1 cup frozen organic strawberries

1 cup orange juice

2 tablespoons Chambord

1 teaspoon fresh lemon juice

1 cup light rum

Strawberry and orange slices,
    for garnish

Preparation:

Fill a highball glass with ice; add the vodka. Combine the remaining ingredients in a blender and purée until smooth. Pour over the vodka and ice. Serve garnished with fresh strawberries and orange slices.

CRANBERRY-GRAPEFRUIT FIZZ

Makes 2 (12-ounce) Drinks

C ranberries, citrus, and pomegranates all have antioxidants, such as vitamin C, that will boost your immunity, especially during cold and flu season. A drink like the one below could become your go-to thirst quencher in the colder months, just be mindful of the alcohol addition.

Ingredients:

1 cup cranberry juice

1 cup grapefruit juice

1 cup sparkling water

Juice of ½ lime

½ cup Prosecco

Preparation:

Combine the ingredients in a large pitcher. Stir, and serve in tall glasses over ice.

LYCHEE COCKTAIL

Makes 1 Serving

I've always liked the subtle tang of lychees, a pitted fruit, or nut, that's got the right amount of neutrally sweet juice balanced with the right amount of acidity.

Ingredients:

2 ounces white wine

1 ounce light rum

1 ounce lychee juice

Dash lime juice

Lime slices, as garnish, optional

Lychee fruit, as garnish, optional

Preparation:

Combine all the ingredients in a cocktail shaker with ice. Shake and strain into a chilled wine glass or champagne flute. Garnish with lime or lychee fruit. If you would like to substitute sparkling wine for the white wine, don't add it to the shaker. Simply mix the other three ingredients and strain into a glass, then top with the sparkling wine.

Any of the previous cocktails can be made just as deliciously, and perhaps more soberly, without the addition of alcohol. That's why we call them mocktails. Following are a few of my favorite nonalcoholic mocktail beverages, which are great for baby showers, luncheons, tea parties, picnics, kids' sport events, in-store events, readings, and more. These are good for your skin because the ingredients are antioxidant rich and bio-available—easily absorbed into the body, providing the best results. Down the hatch!

TART 'N' BUBBLY PUNCH

Makes 12 Servings

T his is my recipe for pretty-in-pink party mocktails. This finished product looks great on a festive table in that massive crystal-cut punch bowl you so rarely use.

Ingredients:

10 to 15 blueberries

6 ounces Acai juice

3 ounces lychee juice

8 cups sugar-free cranberry juice

1 liter cranberry–ginger ale

2 cups crushed ice

Preparation:

Start by filling a small container with water and about 10 to 15 blueberries and freeze in advance. Mix the remaining ingredients together in a large punch bowl slowly adding in the cranberry–ginger ale and crushed ice last. When the punch is ready for presentation and serving, simply crack out your blueberry ice block and add it to the punch bowl.

STRAIGHT-LIME MOJITO

Makes 12 Servings

I like to think of this drink as the amusement park version of a mojito. It's got the refreshing fresh mint and cool sherbet happening, along with good-for-you lime juice and thirst-quenching club soda.

Ingredients:

3 cups water

1½ cups Truvia Baking Blend

2 cups mint leaves

2 cups lime sherbet, softened

1 cup lime juice

8 cups club soda

Lime slices, for garnish

Preparation:

1 Combine 2 cups of the water and the Truvia Baking Blend in a microwave-safe bowl; heat in the microwave on high for 5 minutes. Stir the mint into the water; let stand for 5 minutes.

2 Strain and discard the mint leaves from the syrup; set aside.

3 Stir the lime sherbet, lime juice, and remaining 1 cup of water together in a large pitcher until well combined.

4 Pour the mint-infused syrup into the sherbet mixture. Add the club soda and stir.

5 Serve over ice. Garnish with lime slices.

RUM-FLAVORED POW with COCONUT and SLIVERED ALMONDS

*T*he pow you get from this recipe comes from **p**ineapple, **o**range, and **w**atermelon. These fruits are rich in vitamin C, fiber, folate, magnesium, and potassium. The rum that is called for is an extract, which, depending on the brand you use, may have a small quantity of alcohol in it with a concentrated rum flavor. In general, alcohol in food (for example, Penne a la Vodka, or in recipes that call for "1 cup red wine") is mostly burned off in the cooking process. Therefore, after eating this recipe, or most miniscule-amount-of-alcohol-content recipes, you are safe to drive and operate heavy machinery!

Ingredients:

2 tablespoons Truvia Baking Blend

¼ cup water

Half a lime, juiced

1 teaspoon rum extract

1 cup cubed seedless watermelon

1 cup fresh pineapple chunks

2 medium oranges, peeled and cubed

3 tablespoons coconut

¼ cup slivered almonds

Preparation:

1 In a small saucepan, heat the Truvia Baking Blend in the water until dissolved. Remove from the heat and cool. Add the lime juice and rum extract.

2 Place the fruit in a medium bowl, add the coconut and sugar water. Toss thoroughly. Cover and refrigerate for up to 1 hour to allow the flavors to blend and harmonize (think of this as marinating).

3 Place the fruit mixture in four parfait glasses, top with slivered almonds, and serve.

HONEY-GRAPE DRINK

Makes 2 Servings

*C*hildren love this simple drink. It's a fun one to share at a tea party, just mind the carpet!

Ingredients:

1 cup grape juice

2 tablespoons honey

¼ cup of boiling water

2 tablespoons lemon juice (optional)

Preparation:

Heat 1 cup of grape juice. Set aside.

Mix 2 tablespoons of honey with ¼ cup of boiling water, stir until blended and dissolved, then add enough of the hot grape juice to fill a 12-ounce glass. For variety, 2 tablespoons of lemon juice may be added.

 Honey Facial, Darling

With clean, washed hands, take a few drops of local honey on your fingertip and dab it over any acne. Do this at night before going to bed and keep on overnight. To keep the honey intact on acne, cover the applied surface with small round Band-Aids. In the morning, gently remove the Band-Aids and rinse your face with lukewarm water. If done regularly, this natural solution will help with treating acne scars as well.

BANANA-GRAPE SMOOTHIE

Makes 1 Serving

*T*his is a delicious drink that goes down nicely in the morning when you're short on time but need a blast of nutrients and energy.

Ingredients:

2 large bananas

2 handfuls red seedless grapes

1 cup ice

¼ cup almond milk or soy

Preparation:

Place the bananas and grapes into a blender and mix until it becomes a smooth liquid. Add the ice and blend until crushed. Add the milk, mix until smooth, and pour into a tall glass. Serve.

Conclusion:
How It All Began

People tell me I'm humble. Mostly, I'm a spiritual person whose kindly, tenacious drive and success were inspired by my own devastating skin problems and the terminal illness of my late father. It really all started from there. Hard Work + Courage + Creating an Opportunity = Success. We all have questions, concerns, and secrets about our skin, health, and how to look our best. Hopefully, yours have now been addressed through correcting the challenged areas rather than camouflaging them. But you must remember that you are beautiful, period. This book is just a vehicle to help bring out what is already within you: the even more gorgeous you!

I also know what it feels like to desperately want to improve one's life but not have the financial resources to do so. I grew up of humble means and had to work—a lot, at age fourteen—to even afford my first Neutrogena cleanser, which is so ironic, because I later went on to launch the Neutrogena Men's line (and many other popular products for Johnson & Johnson). Years later, when some money did start coming in from my businesses, I continued to educate myself on how I could empower my skin and not just rely on a bottle of cream, lotions, pills, or potions to do the job for me. I also put myself back into school to become an esthetician so I could understand all sides of the process from the creation of products to the development of protocols (how to use certain ingredients in a series or process), and then I worked with endocrinologists to understand how to best deliver nutrients to the body. I went through all this so I could help my father, myself, and you. I wanted to learn how to heal my skin from the inside out.

Cooking Your Way to Gorgeous is the answer to great skin and improved health, cooking with everyday items and getting the most out of comfort food—with a kick. And now you are a pioneer of this information, too, knowing that, for example, *camu camu* is the next superfood, and that *red palm oil* can power your skin to gorgeous. Innovative health and beauty eating ideas *can* come from uncomplicated recipes where good-tasting

246

food is never sacrificed. It's all about great taste with healthier options. Tell a friend! (P.S. If salt and pepper were the common flavor add-ins in your everyday cooking, notice how this book has turned you on to the health-promoting benefits of numerous spices that can kick up the flavor quotient and benefit skin, too.)

Like you, I will gladly try most any food if I think it may improve my skin. I am a beauty foodie™, but what I eat has to taste good or I simply can't follow through. I know you want to do it all but have limited time, and, now that you have learned how to improve your diet without losing the foods you love, you can really change your life from the inside out! A beautiful change is the best kind of change we can ask for.

If you have learned a thing, or three, from *Cooking Your Way to Gorgeous*, then I feel confident that my work has been done. But since there's always more to do, I am now hard at work on my next book, *Scott-Vincent Borba's Great Starts*.

Lastly, I want to thank you for all your love and support. Being a pioneer is lonely work and most times fraught with challenges. Without you, I wouldn't have made it this far, and, from the bottom of my heart, I sincerely thank you for that. Every day, I make it a point to do something good for someone else. Today I pass that baton to you. Live a beautiful, spiritual life, and share a loving recipe from me with a friend or family member. When they know you are thinking about them and trying to help them live a better, healthier life, it's one of the best feelings in the world.

God bless and besos to you!

Scott-Vincent Borba

Celebrity Esthetician | Nutraceutical Expert

About the Author

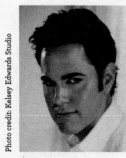

Scott-Vincent Borba has been on the cutting edge of beauty innovation for over two decades, leading the cosmetic industry into the future. His acclaimed background in the beauty industry and his foresight in market development have defined him as an entrepreneur with high merit. As creator and founder of BORBA™, cofounder of e.l.f. cosmetics, and creator and founder of Scott-Vincent Borba Omni Media, Scott-Vincent is posed to change the way people think about skin care.

Scott-Vincent Borba has created a new evolutionary skin-care line that is set to revolutionize beauty and the body, pioneering an emerging category in the marketplace called Nutraceuticals. Independent from any other line or delivery system, BORBA SKIN BALANCE WATER, for example, a technologically advanced Nutraceutical water, improves the overall quality of skin from the inside out. His new company Scott-Vincent Borba, Inc. is his first solo brand. When he launched it on HSN in Fall 2012, the entire line sold out in minutes.

Since graduating with a Bachelor of Science degree from Santa Clara University, he has succeeded as a high-fashion model, TV personality, and, most currently, a licensed celebrity esthetician with the aim of understanding skin on a deeper level and furthering his credentials in that category. Currently, he serves as creative director, and executive vice president of marketing of Toppik, Inc., overseeing product development, retail planning, advertising, social media, and DRTV media campaign.

The youngest of five children, Scott-Vincent was born in a small farming town in Visalia, California. "I received unequivocal guidance and support from my parents," he says. "They encouraged my ambitions to escape the constraints of the small town and create something bigger, something significant of my life."

Scott-Vincent is an active supporter of and global spokesperson for Covenant House California, a nonprofit organization providing food, shelter, life-skills counseling, and education for youth in need. His dedication to the cause is deeply rooted in the belief that when children are provided with the proper mentorship, tools, and spiritual foundation, they will evolve into healthy contributors to society. Scott-Vincent is also a passionate representative for Pancreatic Action Network. Since the passing of his beloved father, he became determined to serve as an advocate for individuals facing this debilitating disease.

Scott-Vincent continues to challenge himself by pursuing additional creative outlets, such as writing, singing, and acting. *Cooking Your Way to Gorgeous* is preceded by his two other bestselling beauty philosophy books—*Makeup for Dummies,* which sold out at Walmarts nationwide, and *Skintervention,* over 15,000 copies sold and counting.

Become part of his family by signing up at Scottvincentborba.com or liking scott-vincentborba on Facebook or SVBorba on Twitter.

About the Writer

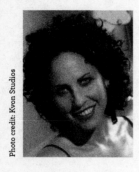

Photo credit: Kvon Studios

Writer **Ali Morra-Pearlman** grew up in Los Angeles, California, and spent her adventurous youth in and around the entertainment industry. She also traveled extensively, studying a variety of cultures and put her divergent experiences and interests to use through a vital journalism career covering health and nutrition, food, travel, city life, cosmetics, and beauty. Her personal features, columns, promotional campaigns, and reviews have appeared in AOL, the *Los Angeles Times, New York Daily News, New York Sun, New York Post, New York Observer, New York Times Sunday Styles, New York Resident, Metro New York, Boston Herald,* and Chicago *RedEye* newspapers, as well as numerous fashion and beauty magazines and websites.

Through her midtwenties, Ali went to work at New York Fashion Week, freelancing for 7th on Sixth "under the tents." and blazed her way from intern to All-Access status, writing fashion features along the way. She also cohosted "Sex and the Single Girl" on AM 640 radio, and contributed a health and wellness relationships-advice column in *amNew York* newspaper. Ali worked as a copywriter for Martha Stewart in promotional and editorial packaging for the Kmart "Everyday" brand; and as senior copywriter for national fashion chain, New York & Company, Ali successfully transitioning the brand image from dowdy to chic.

She is a certified Cambridge English and Berlitz teacher and Boston University alumnus. From maternity modeling to marketing manager for facial plastic surgeon (and husband) Steven J. Pearlman, her interests and abilities are widespread. When not busy raising her five-year-old twin girls, Ali is at work on a collection of steamy short stories. She resides with her family in Westchester County, New York.

Ali met Scott-Vincent on a Los Angeles-New York flight, where their obsession for 'products' was shared and their collaboration was inspired.

Index